Coping with Guilt

Dr Windy Dryden was born in London in 1950. He has worked in psycho-therapy and counselling for over 35 years, and is the author or editor of over 190 books, including *Self-discipline: How to get it and how to keep it* (Sheldon Press, 2009), *Coping with Life's Challenges: Moving on from adversity* (Sheldon Press, 2010), *Coping with Envy* (Sheldon Press, 2010), *How to Develop Inner Strength* (Sheldon Press, 2011), *Coping with Manipulation: When others blame you for their feelings* (Sheldon Press, 2011) and *Transforming Eight Deadly Emotions into Healthy Ones* (Sheldon Press, 2012).

Overcoming Common Problems Series

Selected titles

A full list of titles is available from Sheldon Press,
36 Causton Street, London SW1P 4ST and on our website at
www.sheldonpress.co.uk

101 Questions to Ask Your Doctor
Dr Tom Smith

Asperger Syndrome in Adults
Dr Ruth Searle

The Assertiveness Handbook
Mary Hartley

Assertiveness: Step by step
Dr Windy Dryden and Daniel Constantinou

Backache: What you need to know
Dr David Delvin

Birth Over 35
Sheila Kitzinger

Body Language: What you need to know
David Cohen

Bulimia, Binge-eating and their Treatment
Professor J. Hubert Lacey, Dr Bryony Bamford
and Amy Brown

The Cancer Survivor's Handbook
Dr Terry Priestman

The Chronic Pain Diet Book
Neville Shone

Cider Vinegar
Margaret Hills

Coeliac Disease: What you need to know
Alex Gazzola

**Coping Successfully with Chronic Illness:
Your healing pain**
Neville Shone

Coping Successfully with Pain
Neville Shone

Coping Successfully with Prostate Cancer
Dr Tom Smith

Coping Successfully with Shyness
Margaret Oakes, Professor Robert Bor
Dr Carina Eriksen

Coping Successfully with Ulcerative Colitis
Peter Cartwright

Coping Successfully with Varicose Veins
Christine Craggs-Hinton

Coping Successfully with Your Hiatus Hernia
Dr Tom Smith

Coping When Your Child Has Cerebral Palsy
Jill Eckersley

Coping with Anaemia
Dr Tom Smith

Coping with Asthma in Adults
Mark Greener

**Coping with Birth Trauma and Postnatal
Depression**
Lucy Jolin

Coping with Bowel Cancer
Dr Tom Smith

Coping with Bronchitis and Emphysema
Dr Tom Smith

Coping with Candida
Shirley Trickett

Coping with Chemotherapy
Dr Terry Priestman

Coping with Chronic Fatigue
Trudie Chalder

Coping with Coeliac Disease
Karen Brody

Coping with Diverticulitis
Peter Cartwright

Coping with Drug Problems in the Family
Lucy Jolin

Coping with Dyspraxia
Jill Eckersley

Coping with Early-onset Dementia
Jill Eckersley

Coping with Eating Disorders and Body Image
Christine Craggs-Hinton

Coping with Envy
Dr Windy Dryden

Coping with Gout
Christine Craggs-Hinton

Coping with Headaches and Migraine
Alison Frith

Coping with Heartburn and Reflux
Dr Tom Smith

Coping with Life after Stroke
Dr Mareeni Raymond

**Coping with Life's Challenges: Moving on
from adversity**
Dr Windy Dryden

Overcoming Common Problems Series

Coping with Manipulation: When others blame you for their feelings
Dr Windy Dryden

Coping with Obsessive Compulsive Disorder
Professor Kevin Gournay, Rachel Piper
and Professor Paul Rogers

Coping with Phobias and Panic
Professor Kevin Gournay

Coping with PMS
Dr Farah Ahmed and Dr Emma Cordle

Coping with Polycystic Ovary Syndrome
Christine Craggs-Hinton

Coping with the Psychological Effects of Cancer
Professor Robert Bor, Dr Carina Eriksen
and Ceilidh Stapelkamp

Coping with Radiotherapy
Dr Terry Priestman

Coping with Rheumatism and Arthritis
Dr Keith Souter

Coping with Snoring and Sleep Apnoea
Jill Eckersley

Coping with Stomach Ulcers
Dr Tom Smith

Coping with Suicide
Maggie Helen

Coping with Type 2 Diabetes
Susan Elliot-Wright

Depressive Illness: The curse of the strong
Dr Tim Cantopher

The Diabetes Healing Diet
Mark Greener and Christine Craggs-Hinton

Divorce and Separation: A legal guide for all couples
Dr Mary Welstead

Dying for a Drink
Dr Tim Cantopher

Dynamic Breathing: How to manage your asthma
Dinah Bradley and Tania Clifton-Smith

Epilepsy: Complementary and alternative treatments
Dr Sallie Baxendale

The Fibromyalgia Healing Diet
Christine Craggs-Hinton

Fibromyalgia: Your Treatment Guide
Christine Craggs-Hinton

Free Yourself from Depression
Colin and Margaret Sutherland

A Guide to Anger Management
Mary Hartley

The Heart Attack Survival Guide
Mark Greener

Helping Children Cope with Grief
Rosemary Wells

High-risk Body Size: Take control of your weight
Dr Funké Baffour

How to Beat Worry and Stress
Dr David Delvin

How to Come Out of Your Comfort Zone
Dr Windy Dryden

How to Cope with Difficult People
Alan Houel and Christian Godefroy

How to Develop Inner Strength
Dr Windy Dryden

How to Eat Well When You Have Cancer
Jane Freeman

How to Live with a Control Freak
Barbara Baker

How to Lower Your Blood Pressure: And keep it down
Christine Craggs-Hinton

How to Manage Chronic Fatigue
Christine Craggs-Hinton

The IBS Healing Plan
Theresa Cheung

Let's Stay Together: A guide to lasting relationships
Jane Butterworth

Living with Angina
Dr Tom Smith

Living with Asperger Syndrome
Dr Joan Gomez

Living with Autism
Fiona Marshall

Living with Bipolar Disorder
Dr Neel Burton

Living with Crohn's Disease
Dr Joan Gomez

Living with Eczema
Jill Eckersley

Living with Fibromyalgia
Christine Craggs-Hinton

Living with Gluten Intolerance
Jane Feinmann

Living with IBS
Nuno Ferreira and David T. Gillanders

Living with Loss and Grief
Julia Tugendhat

Living with Osteoarthritis
Dr Patricia Gilbert

Living with Osteoporosis
Dr Joan Gomez

Living with Physical Disability and Amputation
Dr Keren Fisher

Overcoming Common Problems Series

Living with Rheumatoid Arthritis
Philippa Pigache

Living with Schizophrenia
Dr Neel Burton and Dr Phil Davison

Living with a Seriously Ill Child
Dr Jan Aldridge

Living with a Stoma
Professor Craig A. White

Living with Tinnitus and Hyperacusis
Dr Laurence McKenna, Dr David Baguley
and Dr Don McFerran

Losing a Parent
Fiona Marshall

**Making Sense of Trauma: How to tell
your story**
Dr Nigel C. Hunt and Dr Sue McHale

Menopause in Perspective
Philippa Pigache

Motor Neurone Disease: A family affair
Dr David Oliver

The Multiple Sclerosis Diet Book
Tessa Buckley

Natural Treatments for Arthritis
Christine Craggs-Hinton

Osteoporosis: Prevent and treat
Dr Tom Smith

Overcome Your Fear of Flying
Professor Robert Bor, Dr Carina Eriksen
and Margaret Oakes

Overcoming Agoraphobia
Melissa Murphy

Overcoming Anorexia
Professor J. Hubert Lacey, Christine
Craggs-Hinton and Kate Robinson

Overcoming Emotional Abuse
Susan Elliot-Wright

**Overcoming Gambling: A guide for problem
and compulsive gamblers**
Philip Mawer

Overcoming Hurt
Dr Windy Dryden

Overcoming Jealousy
Dr Windy Dryden

Overcoming Loneliness
Alice Muir

**Overcoming Panic and Related Anxiety
Disorders**
Margaret Hawkins

Overcoming Procrastination
Dr Windy Dryden

Overcoming Shyness and Social Anxiety
Dr Ruth Searle

**The Pain Management Handbook:
Your personal guide**
Neville Shone

The Panic Workbook
Dr Carina Eriksen, Professor Robert Bor
and Margaret Oakes

Reducing Your Risk of Dementia
Dr Tom Smith

Self-discipline: How to get it and how to keep it
Dr Windy Dryden

The Self-Esteem Journal
Alison Waines

Sinusitis: Steps to healing
Dr Paul Carson

Stammering: Advice for all ages
Renée Byrne and Louise Wright

Stress-related Illness
Dr Tim Cantopher

Ten Steps to Positive Living
Dr Windy Dryden

**Therapy for Beginners: How to get the best out
of counselling**
Professor Robert Bor, Sheila Gill and Anne Stokes

Think Your Way to Happiness
Dr Windy Dryden and Jack Gordon

**Tranquillizers and Antidepressants: When to
take them, how to stop**
Professor Malcolm Lader

**Transforming Eight Deadly Emotions
into Healthy Ones**
Dr Windy Dryden

The Traveller's Good Health Guide
Dr Ted Lankester

Treating Arthritis Diet Book
Margaret Hills

Treating Arthritis: The drug-free way
Margaret Hills and Christine Horner

Treating Arthritis: More ways to a drug-free life
Margaret Hills

Treating Arthritis: The supplements guide
Julia Davies

Understanding Obsessions and Compulsions
Dr Frank Tallis

Understanding Traumatic Stress
Dr Nigel Hunt and Dr Sue McHale

The User's Guide to the Male Body
Jim Pollard

When Someone You Love Has Dementia
Susan Elliot-Wright

**When Someone You Love Has Depression:
A handbook for family and friends**
Barbara Baker

Coping with Guilt

DR WINDY DRYDEN

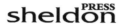
sheldon **PRESS**

First published in Great Britain in 2013

Sheldon Press
36 Causton Street
London SW1P 4ST
www.sheldonpress.co.uk

British Library Cataloguing-in-Publication Data
A catalogue record for this book is available from the British Library

ISBN 978-1-84709-137-6
eBook ISBN 978-1-84709-288-5

Typeset by Caroline Waldron, Wirral, Cheshire
First printed in Great Britain by Ashford Colour Press
Subsequently digitally printed in Great Britain

Produced on paper from sustainable forests

Contents

1 The 'ABCs' of Cognitive Behavioural Therapy   1

2 Understanding guilt   7

3 Understanding remorse: the healthy alternative to guilt   24

4 Preparing the ground for change   37

5 Defining your guilt problem and setting a goal with
   respect to this defined problem   48

6 Assessing a specific example of your guilt problem and
   setting goals with respect to this specific example   57

7 Questioning your beliefs   65

8 Deepening conviction in your remorse-based
   rational beliefs   78

9 Dealing with lapses in guilt and preventing relapse   89

10 How to become less prone to guilt   100

Index   113

1

The 'ABCs' of
Cognitive Behavioural Therapy

Introduction

This book is based on ideas that stem from a tradition in counselling and psychotherapy known as Cognitive Behavioural Therapy (CBT). This tradition has received much attention in the popular and professional press since it is the one that is most frequently recommended for a variety of psychological problems by the National Institute for Health and Clinical Excellence (NICE), whose task is to recommend treatments (both medical and psychological) that have been shown to be effective.

CBT in a nutshell

Cognitive Behavioural Therapy is a therapeutic tradition that focuses particularly on how we think and how we behave in understanding whether we respond healthily or unhealthily to life's adversities. It is a tradition that was founded by two Americans working separately in the 1950s: Dr Albert Ellis, the originator of the first CBT approach known as Rational Emotive Behaviour Therapy, and Dr Aaron Beck, the originator of Cognitive Therapy, perhaps the most practised form of CBT today. This book is based on both approaches and on the works of others in the CBT tradition.

However, while CBT in its present form dates from the 1950s, it has its roots in Stoic philosophy and, in particular, the writings of Epictetus (AD 55–135) whose frequently quoted statement defines the heart of CBT: 'People are disturbed not by things, but by the views which they take of them.' Let's take a closer look at the major principles of CBT.

The 'ABCs' of CBT

CBT employs an 'ABC' model to help people understand how we disturb ourselves about life's adversities. Let me put Epictetus's dictum, presented above, into the 'ABC' framework before I explain this model in more detail:

'A' = things
'B' = view
'C' = disturbance.

There are a number of approaches in the CBT tradition and each one uses the 'ABC' model in a slightly different way. As this book is most closely associated with a CBT approach devised by Dr Albert Ellis, known as Rational Emotive Behaviour Therapy (REBT), I will present REBT's 'ABC' model here:

'A' = adversity
'B' = beliefs
'C' = consequences of the belief about 'A'.

Let me discuss the 'ABC' elements in turn, beginning with 'B' (beliefs) which is the heart of CBT.

'B' stands for beliefs: the heart of CBT

As Epictetus noted all those years ago, the beliefs that we hold about events largely determine how we respond to these events. This, in my opinion, is the heart of CBT. Albert Ellis, the founder of REBT, argued further that the rationality of the beliefs that we hold has a crucial effect on the healthiness of our responses. Let's consider this more closely.

Irrational beliefs underpin unhealthy responses

Albert Ellis argued that irrational beliefs about life's adversities underpin our unhealthy emotional and behavioural responses to these adversities. Here is what Ellis meant by an irrational belief:

An *irrational belief* is:
- rigid or extreme
- false
- illogical
- largely unproductive in its consequences.

Ellis listed four major irrational beliefs:

A rigid belief

When you hold a rigid belief, you focus on what you want or don't want in a given situation, and then you make this desire rigid by demanding that you must get what you want or that you must not get what you don't want.

An awfulizing belief

When you hold an awfulizing belief, you acknowledge that it is bad when your desires are not met, and then you make this extreme by saying that it is awful or the end of the world when you don't get what you want or when you get what you don't want.

A discomfort intolerance belief

When you hold a discomfort intolerance belief, you hold the extreme idea that it is unbearable when your desires are not met.

A depreciation belief

When you hold a depreciation belief about yourself, others and/or life conditions, the following is the case:

* You depreciate yourself when you hold yourself responsible for the adversity that has befallen you.
* You depreciate others when you consider that they are responsible for the adversity that has befallen you.
* You depreciate life conditions when you consider that these are responsible for the adversity that has befallen you.

Rational beliefs underpin healthy responses

Albert Ellis argued that rational beliefs about life's adversities underpin our healthy emotional and behavioural responses to these adversities. Here is what Ellis meant by a rational belief:

A *rational belief* is:

* flexible or non-extreme
* true
* logical
* largely productive in its consequences.

Ellis listed four major rational beliefs:

A flexible belief

When you hold a flexible belief you focus on what you want or don't want in a given situation, and then you keep this desire flexible by acknowledging that you don't have to get what you want or that you don't have to be spared getting what you don't want.

A non-awfulizing belief

When you hold a non-awfulizing belief, you acknowledge that it is bad when your desires are not met, and then you keep this non-extreme by saying that it is not awful or the end of the world when you don't get what you want or when you get what you don't want.

A discomfort tolerance belief

When you hold a discomfort tolerance belief, you hold the non-extreme idea that while it may be difficult for you to put up with the situation where your desires are not met, this is not unbearable and it is worth bearing.

An unconditional acceptance belief

When you hold an unconditional acceptance belief about yourself, others and/or life conditions, the following is the case:

- You accept yourself unconditionally as a complex, unrateable, fallible human being who is largely responsible, in your view, for the adversity that has befallen you.
- You accept others unconditionally as complex, unrateable, fallible human beings who are largely responsible, in your view, for the adversity that has befallen you.
- You accept life conditions unconditionally when you consider that these are responsible for the adversity that has befallen you.

'A' stands for adversity

Because of the nature of this book I will refer to 'A' as an adversity, which is a significantly negative life event. However, when Albert Ellis first introduced his version of the 'ABC' model, 'A' stood for 'activating event'. This was the event that activated the person's beliefs and explained his or her response to the event in question. In this model, 'A' could be something that actually happened (an actual event) or it could be something that the person thought had happened (an inferred event) but which may or may not have happened.

'C' stands for the consequences of the belief about the adversity

There are three major consequences of holding beliefs about life's adversities. These consequences are emotional, behavioural and thinking in nature. Although in reality these consequences are interrelated, I will discuss them separately here.

Emotional consequences

By definition, an adversity is a negative event and therefore it is quite appropriate, and indeed healthy, for you to have negative emotions if you experience such an adversity. Yes, that's right – negative emotions can be healthy. CBT and, in particular, REBT distinguish between emotions that are negative in feeling tone but healthy in effects, and emotions that are negative in feeling tone but unhealthy in effects. The former are known as healthy negative emotions (HNEs) and help you move on when you encounter a life challenge, while the latter are known as unhealthy negative emotions (UNEs), and when you experience these feelings you tend to get stuck or bogged down and don't move on. In this book, guilt is regarded as an unhealthy negative emotion, while its healthy negative emotional alternative is known as remorse.

According to CBT, unhealthy negative emotions largely stem from irrational beliefs about life's adversities while healthy negative emotions largely stem from rational beliefs about these same adversities.

Behavioural consequences

When you hold a belief about an adversity, you act in a certain way or have an urge to act in a certain way which you may or may not put into practice. This latter is called an action tendency in CBT.

According to CBT, unconstructive behaviour and action tendencies largely stem from irrational beliefs about life's adversities, while constructive behaviour and action tendencies stem largely from rational beliefs about these same adversities.

Thinking consequences

So far we have seen that beliefs have an impact on the way you feel about and act in response to an adversity. In addition, your beliefs have an impact on your subsequent thinking that accompanies either your unhealthy negative emotion or your healthy negative emotion about the adversity at 'A'. Thus, when your beliefs are irrational (i.e. rigid and/or extreme) then your subsequent thinking is likely to be grossly distorted and skewed in a negative direction. However, when your beliefs are rational (i.e. flexible and/or non-extreme), your subsequent thinking is likely to be balanced and realistic.

In Chapter 2, I will show you how the 'ABCs' of CBT can shed light on your understanding of guilt. Unless you have a full understanding of this unhealthy negative emotion, you will not be in a good position to change it.

2

Understanding guilt

Before I discuss guilt, a word on terminology. I make the distinction between being guilty and feeling guilty. By *being guilty*, I refer to your responsibility for doing something wrong, for failing to do the right thing or for harming or hurting someone. By *feeling guilty*, I mean the emotion you experience when you blame or condemn yourself for doing something wrong, for failing to do the right thing or for harming or hurting someone. Because it is based on irrational beliefs and generally has disturbed consequences, I consider guilt to be a disturbed negative emotion. A feeling of remorse is a healthy response to doing wrong, etc., because it is based on responsibility without self-blame and generally has healthy consequences, as I will explain more fully later in the book.

In this chapter, I will begin by considering episodic guilt. This refers to the guilt that you experience in specific episodes. Later, I will discuss chronic guilt, which is where you experience guilt in many different situations and where it has a detrimental effect on your life. As you will see, episodic guilt does have a detrimental effect on the way you feel, think and behave, but these effects are limited to the situations in which you experience it. Episodic guilt may, of course, be a specific instance of chronic guilt, and when you experience the latter it is best to begin to deal with it by examining instances of episodic guilt.

How you make yourself feel guilty: general steps

In order for you to feel guilty and stay feeling guilty, you tend to do the following:

- You make a guilt-related inference.
- You bring guilt-based irrational beliefs to that inference.
- You think in ways that are consistent with the above irrational beliefs.
- You act in ways that are consistent with these irrational beliefs.

I will deal with these issues one at a time.

Guilt-related inferences

To feel guilty, you need to make one or more inferences about what is going on in your life. These inferences don't have to be true: the important point is that you think they are true. Here is a list of common guilt-related inferences:

You have broken your moral or ethical code

Here are some examples of this type of guilt-related inference:

- You took stationery from work without asking for permission.
- You cheated on your partner.
- You made racist remarks.

You failed to live up to your moral or ethical code

Here are some examples of this type of guilt-related inference:

- You failed to help someone who required assistance.
- You do not pray every day.
- You did not give to charity.

You have harmed or hurt the feelings of others

Here are some examples of this type of guilt-related inference:

- You forgot your mother's birthday with the result that she felt hurt.
- You told your child off so that she cried.
- You got someone into trouble at work.

You hold and rehearse irrational beliefs about your guilt-related inference

Once again, I want to stress that it is not your guilt-related inference that leads you to feel guilty; rather, at the heart of your feelings of guilt lie a set of irrational beliefs about the inferences that you make. In this context, you will not feel guilty about (1) breaking your moral or ethical code, (2) not living up to your moral or ethical code or (3) harming someone or hurting his or her feelings, without holding irrational beliefs about these inferences.

So let me discuss the irrational beliefs that are at the root of guilt. As discussed in Chapter 1, they take the form of a rigid belief and one of three extreme beliefs about the three guilt-related inferences that I discussed above. In guilt, the extreme belief is most frequently a self-depreciation belief and, as such, I will concentrate on this extreme belief in this book. Now let me expand on this.

Rigid beliefs

As I have shown, when you feel guilt, the essence of this emotion is that you hold and practise guilt-based irrational beliefs. Moreover, I have stressed that these irrational beliefs have two major components: a rigid belief and a self-depreciation belief. A rigid belief is relatively straightforward. It is absolute and comes in the form of a must, absolute should, have to, got to, among others. While it is based on a preference, it is a transformation of that preference into something rigid. As such, it brooks no exception and takes into account no mitigating circumstances.

The major guilt-based negative self-judgements

Self-depreciation beliefs in guilt are derived from rigid beliefs and are a little more varied; here I will outline the major guilt-based negative self-judgements. Before I list these self-depreciation beliefs, remember that a self-depreciation belief involves you making a global negative judgement about yourself. You are not just rating a part of yourself; rather, you are rating the whole of your 'self'.

'I am bad'

The main form of self-depreciation in guilt is 'I am bad'. This is sometimes expressed as 'I am a bad person', 'I am rotten' or 'I am a rotten person'. The hallmark of this form of self-depreciation at the point when you are experiencing guilt is that your entire 'self' is morally corrupt. Most of the time you think this way after you have (1) broken your moral code, (2) failed to live up to your moral code or (3) harmed or hurt someone's feelings, as I have discussed above. When you do so you are making the part–whole error: evaluating your entire 'self' on the basis of one of its parts. In simple terms, you jump from 'It's bad' to 'I'm bad'. For example:

- 'Because I stole stationery from my place of work, I am a bad person.'
- 'Because I failed to give to charity, I am bad.'
- 'Because I hurt my sister's feelings by saying that I didn't like her new dress, I am a rotten person.'

This process of over-generalizing from a part of you to the whole of you is common to virtually all guilt-based negative self-judgements.

'I am less good than I would have been if . . .'

Although you may not condemn yourself entirely you may still make yourself feel guilty (although not as guilty as when you do condemn yourself entirely) by evaluating yourself as less good than you would be if you hadn't done the wrong thing, had done the right thing or hadn't caused harm or hurt to others. For example, if Jack has failed to live up to his moral/ethical code by not giving to charity, he can still make himself feel guilty by believing: 'I absolutely should have given to charity and since I didn't I am less good than I would have been if I had made a charitable donation.'

'I am selfish'

If you experience chronic guilt (i.e. you feel guilty often and across different situations) it is likely that you tend to be selfless and put the interests of others before your own. When you even think of putting your own healthy interests before the interests of others, you feel guilty and back down because you believe: 'I must make sure that others are catered for before I go for what I want, and if I put myself before others then I am a selfish person.'

The following vignette illustrates this dynamic.

Joy was a 44-year-old single woman who was the principal carer for her aging mother, with whom she lived. Joy regularly put her mother's interests before her own, with the result that she rarely went out and had virtually no social life. However, she did have two old school friends who were very loyal to her. These friends badgered Joy incessantly to allow them to take her out to celebrate her 45th birthday, even arranging for a professional carer to look after her mother. Eventually, albeit reluctantly, Joy agreed to go, after obsessively checking with her mother that she didn't mind. However, just before going to the posh restaurant that her friends had booked for the celebration, Joy made herself feel severely guilty and made her apologies before rushing home to her mother. Joy did this because she held the following belief: 'I must not enjoy myself when I know that my mother is not enjoying herself. Because I am putting my pleasure before my mother's feelings I am a selfish person.'

People like Joy shuttle between two positions: selflessness and selfishness. When you do this, you are basically saying that either you put other people's interests before your own or you are a selfish person. What often fuels this belief is your idea that you are unimportant, and the only way that you can gain a sense of importance is by ensuring that you help others achieve their goals or ensure that they don't get upset. Such an idea results in you becoming highly susceptible to others manipulating you through guilt. Thus, Joy's mother successfully manipulated Joy by saying things like: 'Don't worry about me, dear, I'll be all right,' while giving her a pained expression. What this really meant, as Joy fully realized, was: 'I'll be upset if you go out and it will be all your fault.'

When you believe that you are a selfish person, you are doing three things:

- You acknowledge that your behaviour is selfish. It often isn't, but you infer that it is.
- You assume that because you have acted selfishly, you score highly on the trait known as 'selfishness'.
- You use that trait description to define yourself. It is as if you are saying: 'Because I have acted selfishly, I have selfishness and I am therefore a selfish person.' Once you habitually make this 'behaviour → trait → self' translation process, you skip the middle step and define your 'self' on the basis of your behaviour (behaviour → self), e.g. 'Because I acted selfishly I am a selfish person.'

Finally, when you believe that you are a selfish person, most of the time you are implying (although you do not make this explicit) that you are a bad person or at least less good than you would be if you scored highly on selflessness or acted selflessly.

'I don't deserve good things to happen to me. I only deserve bad things'

Another way that you can make yourself feel unhealthily guilty is to consider yourself undeserving of good things, but deserving of bad. This is a more subtle form of self-depreciation and thus more difficult to identify. But if you feel guilty and can't recognize the other forms of guilt-based self-depreciation in your guilt, then you may well resonate with this one.

Inferences at 'A' x irrational beliefs at 'B' = guilt at 'C'

Having discussed the two main irrational beliefs that underpin guilt, let me show how holding such beliefs about each of the three main inferences that I have already discussed in this chapter leads to guilt. In doing so, I will outline a general irrational belief and illustrate it with a specific example.

Guilt about breaking a moral or ethical code

In general, in order to feel guilty about breaking a moral or ethical code, you need to hold a rigid belief about such a code violation (e.g. 'I must not break my moral or ethical code') and a self-depreciation belief about it (e.g. '. . . and because I have broken it, I am a bad person'). For example, one of Carla's moral rules was that it is wrong to criticize one of her friends to another friend. On one occasion, she was annoyed with one of her friends and badmouthed that friend to another friend. Carla made herself guilty about her code violation by holding the following guilt-based irrational belief: 'I absolutely should not have badmouthed my friend and because I did I am a bad person.'

Guilt about not living up to a moral or ethical code

The difference between this situation and the above is that in the above you have committed a 'sin'[1] (known as the sin of commission), i.e. you have done the wrong thing. Here, you have failed to do the right thing (known as the sin of omission). In general, in order to feel guilty about failing to live up to a moral or ethical code, you again tend to hold a rigid belief about such a failure (e.g. 'I must live up to my moral or ethical code') and a consequent self-depreciation belief (e.g. '. . . and because I have not, I am a bad person'). For example, Jack thinks that giving to charity is the right thing to do. One morning, Jack was walking down the road and a street charity worker approached him for a donation. Given that he was in a hurry, Jack refused. From his frame of reference he failed to live up to his ethical code. To feel guilty about his behaviour, Jack brought to the incident the following guilt-based irrational belief: 'I absolutely should have given a donation and because I didn't I am a bad person.'

Guilt about harming or hurting the feelings of someone else

In general, in order to feel guilty about harming or hurting the feelings of someone else, you tend to hold a rigid belief about your role in this situation (e.g. 'I absolutely should not harm or hurt someone') and a self-depreciation about your role (e.g. '. . . and because I did I am a bad person').

For example, Linda wanted to visit her parents over Easter, while her partner wanted to visit his parents in a different part of the country. They ended up seeing her parents, and Linda felt guilty about this situation by first thinking: 'My partner is upset about not seeing his parents and I am the cause of his upset' and then by holding the following guilt-based irrational belief: 'I upset him, which I must not do, and this proves what a bad, selfish person I am.'

Another way for Linda to practise this guilt-based irrational belief in this situation, but this time without feeling guilty (I call this a way of rehearsing emotional disturbance without feeling it), is for her to go along with her partner's wishes. She would do so because (1) she thinks that he would be upset about not seeing his parents and, more

---

1 Whenever I refer to 'sin' in this book, I mean it as shorthand to cover situations where you have (or think you have) (1) broken your moral code, (2) failed to live up to your moral code or (3) hurt someone's feelings.

importantly, (2) she would make herself feel guilty about this because she would hold the following guilt-producing irrational belief: 'If we went to see my parents, I know that he would be upset and I would be the cause of this. I must not upset my partner and I am a bad, selfish person if I do.'

Of course, by going to see his parents, Linda would also have made herself feel guilty about causing her parents' upset about not seeing her. This example shows very clearly that with guilt you are damned whatever you decide to do!

Thinking that stems from guilt-based irrational beliefs

When you hold a guilt-based irrational belief about thinking that you have (1) broken your moral/ethical code, (2) failed to do the right thing and/or (3) caused harm or hurt to others, this belief will influence the way that you subsequently think, as discussed below.

You exaggerate the badness of your behaviour in your mind

Once you have made yourself feel guilty about your 'sin', you tend to think about what you did in exaggerated ways. In particular, you may think that your actions are much worse than when you first focused on them.

Thus, Brenda first made herself feel guilty about hurting her parents' feelings by refusing to do their shopping for them. She then exaggerated this by showing herself that her actions were despicably selfish. Having exaggerated the badness of her behaviour in this way, Brenda then brought a further guilt-inducing irrational belief to this exaggeration, thus making herself even more guilty.

You exaggerate the negative consequences of your behaviour and minimize its positive consequences

Once you have made yourself feel guilty about your 'sin', you exaggerate the negative consequences of your behaviour and minimize its positive consequences.

Thus, Victor made himself feel guilty about stealing stationery from work. Having done so, he thought that he was bound to be caught and that when he was, he would be fired and would find it difficult to get another job (exaggerating the negative consequences of his behaviour). He edited out what he could productively learn from this episode, i.e. that he stole it because he thought he needed it and that he could challenge the belief that he must have what he wants (minimizing the positive consequences of his behaviour).

You assume more personal responsibility for what happened and assign less responsibility to others than the situation warrants

Once you have made yourself feel guilty and you look back on your 'sin' and all the factors involved, you tend to assume far more responsibility than the situation warrants and to assign far less responsibility to relevant others. In a phrase, you think that it is all your fault.

In addition, you keep your feelings of guilt alive by editing out of the picture the responsibility that others have for their own feelings. You do this when you think that you can hurt other people's feelings. Actually, you cannot hurt their feelings. You can treat people badly and harm them physically or materially, but you can't hurt their feelings since they have the choice whether or not to disturb themselves or not about your behaviour towards them.

You engage in 'if only' thinking

'If only' thinking serves to perpetuate guilt after you have begun to experience this emotion.

For example, in good faith Mark made a business decision which unfortunately did not work out, with the result that he had to sack two of his employees to ensure that his company continued trading. He made himself feel guilty by believing that he absolutely should not have acted in a way that had such bad consequences and that he was a bad person because he did so. Mark unwittingly maintained his guilt feelings by showing himself that if only he hadn't acted in that way then he would not have had to sack his two employees. This reinforces Mark's idea that he alone was responsible for sacking his employees. Of course, it may be true that if Mark hadn't made the decision then the two employees would not have lost their jobs. However, it could equally be true that if Mark hadn't made the decision other bad things would have happened.

However, under the influence of his guilt, Mark thought that this bad outcome would not have happened if he hadn't made the decision, and that a good outcome would have happened if he had made a different decision. In doing so, he gave himself a double dose of guilt. First, he made himself feel guilty for taking sole responsibility for the bad outcome ('I am a bad person because I made a decision that resulted in me having to sack two of my employees. I absolutely should not have made such a bad decision'). Second, he made himself feel guilty for not making a different, more effective decision ('If only I had made that other investment that I was considering at the time, then I would not have had to lay off my two employees and things would have flourished. I am a bad person for not making the right decision, as I absolutely should have done').

You judge what you did with the benefit of hindsight only

One of the things that people who do not make themselves feel unhealthily guilty do is to look back at their 'sin' from the perspective of when they took action. Thus, they are able to say: 'Yes, I now see that I broke my moral code, but I was so fixated on getting what I wanted, it did not occur to me that I was breaking my moral code. What I have learned from this situation is that I need to deal with my tendency to become fixated so that I can be more aware of the implications of my behaviour.' In contrast, if you often experience guilt, you don't do this. Rather, you only judge your behaviour with the benefit of hindsight (e.g. 'I could have foreseen what I was going to do and therefore I absolutely should have done so' or 'I now see that it would have been better to do x rather than y, and therefore I absolutely should have done x'). As you can see, hindsight thinking stems from absolute thinking and together they make a very powerful guilt-inducing cocktail. In short, you believe: 'Because I could have done things differently, I absolutely should have done things differently.'

You do not take into account mitigating factors or show yourself compassion

Once you have made yourself feel guilty, you will tend to discount what might be called mitigating factors, i.e. genuine reasons for your behaviour that may help you to take an understanding, compassionate view of your 'sin'. Colloquially, this is often referred to as you 'being hard on yourself'. If you believe that you absolutely should not have broken your moral code, such rigidity precludes you from understanding aspects of the situation that may have prompted you to act as you did. This is why I say that guilt and the rigid beliefs on which it is based are the enemies of compassionate self-understanding.

You fail to appreciate the complexity of the situation

When you do something wrong, for example, you can best view your behaviour from a complex perspective. However, when you feel guilt, you fail to do so.

Thus, when Esther let down her friend, she in fact faced a choice between letting down her friend and letting down her parents. She decided to let down her friend because she thought that it was the lesser of the two evils. However, because Esther held the rigid belief: 'I must not let down people I care about', she looked at this situation in black-and-white terms that failed to appreciate the complexity of the situation in which she found herself. Thus, she concluded: 'Letting down my friend was just plain wrong and that's the end of it. It cannot be justified.'

You think that you will receive due retribution for your behaviour

As I have already discussed, when you make yourself feel guilty, one of the guilt-inducing irrational beliefs that you hold is that you are a bad person. When you hold this belief, it encourages you to infer that bad things will happen to you because you think that you deserve retribution for being a bad person. In short, you believe that bad things happen to bad people because they deserve punishment.

Behaviour that stems from guilt-based irrational beliefs

When you hold guilt-based irrational beliefs, you will tend to act in certain ways. It is important to note that many of these behaviours are both an expression of guilt and an attempt by you to avoid the pain of these feelings. The main point is that these behaviours stem from your guilt-based irrational beliefs and, when you engage in them, help to strengthen your conviction in these beliefs. As such, engaging in guilt-based behaviours renders you more vulnerable to experiencing guilt.

You confess regardless of the consequences

Some say that confession is good for the soul, and this may be the case if you think carefully about the consequences of your confession and judge that it will do you more good than harm. However, if you are prone to guilt you believe that you have to confess your 'sin' to the people involved regardless of the consequences. In doing so, you will strengthen your guilt-based irrational belief: 'I am a bad person and I must unburden myself to become good again.' Of course, confession (outside a religious context) doesn't lead you to become good again and there is every chance that the consequences of your confession will be harmful to you and the other(s) involved. This latter point demonstrates how you can give yourself a double dose of guilt: 'I am a bad person for doing what I did in the first place and a bad person for upsetting the other(s) by confessing my sin in the second place.' So, thoughtless confession will, in all probability, lead you further down the guilt road.

You beg for forgiveness

Another way that you may unwittingly strengthen your guilt-based irrational beliefs is to beg for forgiveness from the other person that you have wronged, harmed or hurt. In begging, rather than asking, for forgiveness, you tend to deepen your conviction that you are a bad, despicable creature who can only be raised up if the other person forgives you. Within this framework, if you are not forgiven you remain a bad person in your mind. If you are forgiven you feel better temporarily, but since your conviction in your badness remains unchecked, you need frequent reassurance that the other has still forgiven you. You thus frequently seek reassurance from this other person that you are still forgiven.

You promise unrealistically not to 'sin' again

After you have wronged, harmed or hurt someone and you have made yourself feel guilty about doing so, one way in which you attempt to make yourself feel better in the short term is to promise the other person that you will not 'sin' again. If the other person accepts your promise you will feel relieved, but in all probability you won't take steps to put your promise into practice by seeking help to address the factors that led you to 'sin' in the first place. Consequently, you will probably 'sin' again if you encounter these factors, and if you do you will probably make yourself feel guilty for your behaviour all over again. On the other hand, if the other person does not accept your promise, you will not gain this short-term relief and will continue to make yourself feel guilty about your 'sin'.

You deprive yourself

When you have made yourself feel guilty, you tend to think that you don't deserve any good things in life. To reinforce this view, you deprive yourself of the good things in life. You may not see your friends, for example, and may not engage in any pleasurable activities. In doing so, you implicitly rehearse the view that the reason you are depriving yourself is that as a person you do not deserve such pleasure because of your 'sin'.

You punish yourself

A more extreme version of depriving yourself is punishing yourself. Here, you are not just saying that you do not deserve good things in your life, you are also saying that you deserve bad things in your life. Consequently, you tend to actively seek out such bad things. For example, you may seek out and spend time with people who actively dislike you or you may engage in tasks that you actively dislike. In doing so, you are acting on the belief that because of your 'sin' you deserve to be treated badly by people who dislike you and you are only fit to engage in tasks that you hate.

You undertake a penance

When you punish yourself for your 'sin', you are in effect saying that because you are bad you deserve to experience bad things. However, when you do penance for your 'sin' (e.g. by deliberately undertaking something onerous) you are saying that you can redeem yourself from your badness by your penance. In doing so, you still hold and unwittingly strengthen the belief that you are a bad person for your 'sin'.

You disclaim responsibility

When you have done something wrong, have failed to do the right thing or have caused harm or hurt to someone and you hold a guilt-inducing irrational belief about your 'sin', you will tend to make yourself guilty. I say 'tend to' here because you can still stop yourself from feeling guilty before guilt takes a hold. You can do this by disclaiming responsibility for your actions. Basically, you can do this in two ways. First, you can place the responsibility on some external factor. This might be another person (e.g. 'Yes, I did let you down, but it was my brother's fault. He made me do it') or some aspect of the environment (e.g. 'I would have helped you out, but the train was delayed'). Second, you can place the responsibility on some internal factor like illness or medication (e.g. 'I don't know what came over me. It must have been the medication I am on'). While you will not actually experience feelings of guilt if you disclaim responsibility in these ways, you are still rehearsing your guilt-inducing irrational beliefs, albeit implicitly.

For example, when Sam tries to convince himself that the reason he let down his friend was due to his brother he is implicitly saying: 'If I acknowledge that I was responsible for letting the other person down, then I would be a bad person. Therefore, to stop blaming myself, I will blame someone else.'

You overcompensate in your behaviour for feelings of guilt

Another way of coping with feelings of guilt is to overcompensate for them. This involves you doing the very opposite of what you feel guilty about. However, when you do this it does result in strengthening your guilt-inducing irrational belief.

Thus, Fay believes that she is a bad person for having upset her friend. She overcompensated for her guilt feelings by going out of her way to be nice to people. She did that because she thought that the only way that she could get away from the belief that she is bad was by doing good. However, in doing so, she unwittingly strengthened the idea that her moral worth as a person is based on the way she treats others. This exemplifies the conditional philosophy of guilt: 'I am bad if I treat others badly. I am good if I treat others well.'

You try to get reassurance from others, but fail to be reassured

After you have made yourself feel guilty for your 'sin', you may be tempted to ask people for reassurance that what you did wasn't wrong, that there was a good reason for what you did, or that you were not really responsible for your actions. It is likely that you will find plenty of people to give you such reassurance, but you won't stay reassured for long. Believing that you are a bad person for doing what you absolutely should not have done means that you are not reassurable, even if an army of volunteers are recruited to reassure you. It will only take one person to say that what you did was wrong and your guilt-inducing irrational belief will lead you back to: 'But it was wrong' and from there to 'Since it was wrong, I absolutely should not have done it, and because I did, I am a bad person.'

The same process happens when another person convinces you, for the moment, that there was good reason for what you did or that you weren't really responsible for your actions. Here, as before, your guilt-inducing irrational belief will lead you to go back and say to yourself: 'But there really wasn't a good reason for my behaviour' or 'But I am responsible for my actions.' When you do go back, you will then feel guilty because you will bring your guilt-inducing irrational belief to these inferences.

You reject offers of forgiveness

I mentioned earlier in this section that when you hold a set of guilt-based irrational beliefs you may tend to beg others for forgiveness. Paradoxically, if you are forgiven, these same beliefs may lead you to reject the very forgiveness that you have begged for. Why? Because when you feel guilty, you think you are bad. You are then desperate to feel better and think that this can be achieved by being forgiven. However, when you are forgiven you may still think that you are a bad person who is not worthy of forgiveness, which you then reject.

When your guilt is chronic

When your guilt is chronic then you experience this emotion much of the time, you are easily manipulated by others, you fail to stand up for yourself, you fail to practise self-care and you think that you are responsible for others' feelings. I now discuss each of these features in turn.

You feel guilty much of the time

If you are particularly prone to guilt you will think that you often do the wrong thing, fail to do the right thing or hurt the feelings of others.

You do this because you hold the following belief, which I call a 'chronic guilt-based general irrational belief':

Whenever I am involved, I must make sure that nothing bad happens or others' feelings are not hurt. If I don't, and bad things happen and/or others are upset, then it is all my fault and I am a bad person.

You then take this belief to relevant situations and, even where your involvement is minimal, you think that you are at fault if there is or may be a bad outcome. As a result you constantly think that you are responsible for any negative outcomes that happen or might happen and end up blaming yourself.

Let me give you a concrete example. Josie had the following chronic guilt-related general irrational belief: 'If I have had dealings with people, I must know that others are not upset in any way as a result. If they are upset, it is my fault and I am a bad person. If I am unsure about how they feel, then I assume that they are upset and I am again the cause, in which case I am a bad person.' She took this belief to a specific situation where her mother asked her over for dinner and Josie said no because she was going out with a friend that night. She explained this to her mother but was not sure of the latter's reaction. Her chronic guilt-based general irrational belief led her to infer that she had upset her mother. It was as if Josie reasoned: 'Because I can't convince myself that I didn't upset my mother, therefore I did.' Her belief did not allow her to think that her mother was probably accepting of her not going to dinner.

Once Josie created her inference, she made herself feel guilty about it by holding a specific version of her chronic guilt-based general irrational belief: 'I upset my mother by turning down her dinner invitation. I absolutely should not have upset my mother in this way and I am a bad person because I did.' Having made herself feel guilty in this way, Josie then thought and acted in ways that were consistent with her guilt-based irrational belief, which had the effect of strengthening this belief.

More generally, Josie experienced guilt whenever others did not show that they were happy in their interactions with her. Her general irrational belief led her (1) to transform her doubt into the inference that she had upset the other person and (2) to think of herself as bad for upsetting them, something she believed she must not do.

You are easily manipulated by others

When you have a chronic problem with guilt, then you are easily manipulated by others. If such people want you to do something for them, for example, all they have to do is to imply that they will be upset if you don't do it and this will lead you to do what you don't particularly want to do.

This phenomenon relies on implicit communication, which I will make explicit in the following example. Kerry's mother was very adept at manipulating her daughter by doing the following. Whenever Kerry wanted to go out but her mother did not want her to, her mother would complain of having chest pains, but would tell her to go out without meaning it. Kerry's mother's implicit communication to her daughter was as follows: 'If you go out, I will have a heart attack and this will be your fault. This will prove that you are bad.' Kerry implicitly responded to this communication as follows: 'If I go out, my mother will have a heart attack and it will be all my fault. This will prove that I am bad.' In other words, Kerry accepted her mother's version of the truth on all three accounts: (1) 'My mother will have a heart attack'; (2) 'If she does it will be all my fault'; and (3) 'It will prove that I am bad.'

This shows if you suffer from with chronic guilt you tend to accept 'reality' as defined by others, particularly when it is being implied that you have done the wrong thing, failed to do the right thing or hurt others' feelings. Also, you may well think that others are making such implications even when they are not doing so.

You fail to stand up for yourself

If you have a chronic guilt problem then you may not stand up for yourself when it is healthy for you to do so. As a result, you tend to have more negative events to deal with than people who do assert themselves. For example, in a work setting you tend to get saddled with work that nobody else wants, and you will tend to work longer hours than others. Why don't you assert yourself? You fail to do so for two reasons. First, you tend to think that if you stand up for yourself others will be upset with you and you will hold yourself responsible for upsetting them. Then you make yourself feel guilty as a result because of the irrational beliefs you hold about upsetting others. Rather than risk upsetting others, then, you decide not to stand up for yourself.

Second, you tend to believe that you need others' approval, and thus if you stand up for yourself you predict others will disapprove of you, which will prove in your mind that you are worthless. In order to avoid thinking that you are worthless you decide, again, not to stand up for yourself.

You fail to practise self-care

If you have a problem with chronic guilt then it is likely that you tend to put the interests of others ahead of your own. You do this for two reasons. First, you think that putting your own interests ahead of those of others means that you are being selfish, and if you are being selfish then this means that you are a bad person. Second, you think that selflessness is a virtue, and thus by putting others first you are being good.

All this means that you fail to practise self-care. Indeed, because you see the world in black-and-white terms, in that you are either being selfless or you are being selfish, you do not even have a 'slot' in your mind for healthy self-care. And if you don't conceptualize self-care, you are hardly likely to practise it. The consequences of failing to look after your own interests can be serious for both your physical and mental well-being in that you will tend to neglect signs that all is not well with you.

You think that you are responsible for others' upset feelings

As I outlined in Chapter 1, this book is based on the principles of Cognitive Behavioural Therapy. Perhaps the most important of these principles when understanding guilt is that this emotion (together with other unhealthy negative emotions) is based on you making certain kinds of inferences and holding a set of rigid and extreme beliefs about these inferences. From this perspective, your feelings are based largely on your thoughts. This is known as the principle of emotional responsibility. If this is true for your feelings then it is also true of others' feelings. Their feelings, therefore, are based largely on the thoughts (inferences and beliefs) that they have about what you have done or not done.

However, if you have a chronic problem with guilt, then you have a very different view on what determines other people's hurt feelings when you are involved. You believe that you are responsible for their hurt feelings. Now, of course, when others feel hurt about what you have done, you contribute to their feelings. This is known as 'A' in the 'ABC' framework described in Chapter 1. But when you take responsibility for others' feelings you argue that 'A' causes 'C'. This is at variance with the 'ABC' model, which states that when others feel hurt (at 'C') about what you have done or failed to do (at 'A') their hurt feelings are largely determined by their own thoughts (at 'B') about 'A'.

Even when the 'ABC' model is explained to you, you will tend to disregard it because of the chronic guilt-based general irrational belief that you hold about others' feelings (e.g. 'When I am involved with others I must make sure that they are not upset. If they are, or there is a chance that they are, then I am responsible for their feelings'). Unless you change this belief, you will continue to take responsibility for the hurt feelings of others.

In the following chapter, I will help you to understand remorse, which is seen in CBT as the healthy alternative to guilt when you have 'sinned'.

3

Understanding remorse: the healthy alternative to guilt

As humans, we do not live in an emotional vacuum. Thus, if you recognize that you have a problem with guilt when you think that you have broken or failed to live up to your moral code or when you think you have hurt someone's feelings, then you need to have a clear vision of what would be healthier for you to feel instead. As I noted at the beginning of Chapter 2, the healthy alternative to guilt is remorse. If you don't have a clear idea of this alternative and think that you should not feel anything or that you should feel less guilty, then you will go back to guilt for the simple reason that you don't know what to aim for instead. Remorse provides a clear alternative to guilt.

In this chapter, I will expand on this point and will (1) detail the inferences that you make when you experience remorse, (2) specify the rational beliefs that underpin remorse and (3) discuss the thoughts and behaviours that often accompany this healthy alternative to guilt.

In the previous chapter, I began by considering episodic guilt and went on to consider chronic guilt. I will follow this structure in this chapter. Initially, I will consider what might be called episodic remorse, which refers to the remorse that you experience in specific episodes. Later, I will discuss what it means to be less prone to guilt and will outline the differences between chronic guilt and what I call 'realistic remorse'.

Understanding the dynamics of remorse

When you feel remorse you tend to do the following:

1 You make an inference.
2 You bring remorse-based rational beliefs to that inference.
3 You think in ways that are consistent with the above rational beliefs.
4 You act in ways that are consistent with these rational beliefs.

I will deal with these issues one at a time.

Remorse-related inferences

When you feel remorse, you actually make the same inferences as you do when you feel guilt. Again, these inferences don't have to be true; the important point is that you think that they are true. Let me remind you what these inferences are:

You have broken your moral or ethical code

Here are some examples of this type of inference. They are the same as in the corresponding section on guilt in Chapter 2 (see p. 8).

- You took stationery from work without asking for permission.
- You cheated on your partner.
- You made racist remarks.

You failed to live up to your moral or ethical code

Here are some examples of this type of inference. They are again the same as in the corresponding section on guilt in Chapter 2 (see p. 8).

- You failed to help someone who required assistance.
- You do not pray every day.
- You did not give to charity.

You have harmed or hurt the feelings of others

Here are some examples of this type of inference. Once again, they are the same as in the corresponding section on guilt in Chapter 2 (see p. 8).

- You forgot your mother's birthday with the result that she felt hurt.
- You told your child off so that she cried.
- You got someone into trouble at work.

The important point to take away from this discussion is this: since the inferences that you make at 'A' in the 'ABC' framework are the same, then working towards feeling remorse rather than guilt must involve changing some other process and not changing your inferences at 'A'.[1]

---

1 It is appropriate to change your inference when it is distorted, but this is not a long-term approach to deal with guilt which stems largely from irrational beliefs, as discussed in Chapter 2.

Rational beliefs underpin remorse

As with guilt, it is not the inference that you made at 'A' that leads to your feelings of remorse at 'C'. Rather, at the heart of your feelings of remorse lies a set of rational beliefs about the inference that you made. In this context, you will feel remorse rather than guilt about (1) breaking your moral or ethical code, (2) not living up to your moral or ethical code or (3) harming someone or hurting their feelings, when the beliefs that you hold about these inferences are rational rather than irrational.

So let me discuss the rational beliefs that are at the root of remorse. As discussed in Chapter 1, they take the form of a flexible belief and one of three non-extreme beliefs about the three listed inferences. In remorse, the non-extreme belief is most frequently an unconditional self-acceptance belief and, as such, I will concentrate on this non-extreme belief in this book. Now let me expand on this.

Flexible beliefs

As I have shown, when you feel remorse the essence of this emotion is that you hold and practise a set of rational beliefs. Moreover, I have stressed that these rational beliefs have two major components: a flexible belief and an unconditional self-acceptance belief. A flexible belief has two components. Like a rigid belief it is based on a preference, but unlike that rigid belief a flexible belief does not transform that preference into something rigid. Indeed, it makes quite clear that it is not rigid. It thus allows for exceptions to the rule and takes into account mitigating circumstances.

Remorse-based unconditional self-acceptance beliefs

Unconditional self-acceptance beliefs in remorse are derived from flexible beliefs and are based on three principles:

1 As a person, you cannot legitimately be given or give yourself a single global rating that defines your essence and your worth, as far as you have it, since you are far too complex and you are constantly in flux.
2 Your worth, as far as you have it, is not dependent upon conditions that change. Thus, your worth stays the same whether or not you break your moral code.
3 It makes sense for you to rate discrete aspects of yourself and your experiences, but it does not make sense to rate your 'self' on the basis of these discrete aspects.

When referring to the concept of human worth above I used the term 'as far as you have it'. There are two versions of an unconditional self-acceptance (USA) belief – one based on worth and one not. When using the concept of worth in an unconditional self-acceptance belief, the most important principle is the unconditional nature of the belief, as in 'I am worthwhile even though I hurt my mother's feelings.' When you choose not to use the concept of worth in a USA belief, you acknowledge the facts about yourself, as in 'I am a fallible, unrateable, ever-changing person even though I hurt my mother's feelings.' Again, note the unconditional nature of this belief.

You may find yourself resisting using USA beliefs because you think that it lets you off the hook concerning your act of commission or omission or the behaviour that resulted in others being hurt. Nothing could be further from the truth. When you hold a USA belief, you accept yourself *and* you take full responsibility for your behaviour – something which people who are psychopathic fail to do.

Inferences at 'A' x rational beliefs at 'B' = remorse at 'C'

Having discussed the two main rational beliefs that underpin guilt, let me show how holding such beliefs about each of the three main inferences that I have already discussed in this chapter leads to remorse. In doing so, I will outline a general rational belief and illustrate it with a specific example.

Remorse about breaking a moral or ethical code

When you feel remorse, but not guilt, about breaking a moral or ethical code, you need to hold a flexible belief about such a code violation (e.g. 'I would much prefer not to break my moral or ethical code, but that does not mean that I must not do so') and an unconditional self-acceptance belief about it (e.g. '. . . I am not a bad person for breaking it. Rather, I am a fallible human being who did the wrong thing'). Carla, who we first met in Chapter 2, broke one of her moral rules by badmouthing one friend to another. She was able to feel remorse, but not guilt, about this code violation by holding and practising the following remorse-based rational belief: 'I really wish that I had not badmouthed my friend, but I am not immune from doing so and nor do I have to be thus immune. I am not a bad person for doing so. I am a complex, fallible human being who did the wrong thing.'

Remorse about not living up to a moral or ethical code

In general, in order to feel remorse, but not guilt, about failing to live up to a moral or ethical code, you again need to hold a flexible belief about such a failure (e.g. 'I would much prefer to live up to my moral or ethical code, but sadly I do not have to do so') and a consequent unconditional self-acceptance belief (e.g. '. . . if I don't, I'm not a bad person, but a fallible, complex human being who has failed to do the right thing').

For example, if you remember, Jack thought that giving to charity was the right thing to do, but he failed to give a donation on one occasion because he was in a hurry. From his frame of reference he failed to live up to his ethical code. To feel remorseful, but not guilty, about his behaviour, Jack would have had to hold the following rational belief: 'I really wish that I had given a donation, but unfortunately there is no law of the universe decreeing that I absolutely should have done so. I am not bad person for failing to do so. Rather, I am a fallible person who failed on this occasion to do the right thing.'

Remorse about harming or hurting the feelings of someone else

In general, in order to feel remorseful, but not guilty, about harming or hurting the feelings of someone else, you once again need to hold both a flexible belief and an unconditional self-acceptance belief about your role in this situation (e.g. 'I really don't want to harm or hurt someone, but I am not immune from doing so and nor do I have to have such immunity. I am not a bad person if I do so. Rather, I am a complex, unrateable, fallible human being').

Linda felt remorse for upsetting her partner when they decided to go to visit her parents rather than his. She was able to feel remorse rather than guilt because she held the following rational belief: 'My partner is upset about not seeing his parents and I am the cause of his upset. I wish I had not upset him, but sadly that does not mean that I must not do so. I am not a bad selfish person, but a fallible human being who upset him on this occasion.'

Thinking that stems from remorse-based rational beliefs

When you hold a remorse-based rational belief about thinking that (1) you have broken your moral code, (2) you have failed to do the right thing and/or (3) you have caused harm or hurt to others, this belief will influence the way that you subsequently think, as discussed below.

You take into account all relevant data when judging whether or not you have 'sinned'

Once you feel remorseful, but not guilty, about your 'sin', you are able to stand back and think about all the factors that are relevant in judging whether or not you have 'sinned'. This is particularly useful if your first response is that you have 'sinned'. If you recall, Brenda made herself guilt about hurting her parents' feelings by refusing to do their shopping for them. When she felt remorseful rather than guilty about this, she was able to see the following: (1) her parents were capable of doing their own shopping; (2) by putting herself first she was caring for herself rather than being selfish; and (3) her parents were using their 'upset' to manipulate her by trying to make her feel bad.

You assume an appropriate level of personal responsibility to self and others

When you feel remorse rather than guilt and you look back on your 'sin' and all the factors involved, you tend to assume an appropriate amount of responsibility, as the situation warrants, and also to assign an appropriate amount of responsibility to relevant others. You do not think that it is all your fault.

In addition, when you feel remorse, you acknowledge that others involved have responsibility for their own feelings. While you recognize that you can't really hurt others' feelings, you do appreciate that you can contribute to their hurt by your behaviour, for which you take full responsibility but without self-blame.

You take into account mitigating factors

If you hold remorse-based rational beliefs, you are prepared to take into account mitigating factors, i.e. genuine reasons for your behaviour that may help you take an understanding, compassionate view of your 'sin'. Colloquially, this is often referred to as you 'being compassionate with yourself' and stands in stark contrast with you 'being hard on yourself' when you hold guilt-based irrational beliefs.

You put your behaviour into an overall context

When you do something wrong, for example, you can best view your behaviour from a complex perspective. Holding a set of remorse-based rational beliefs allows you to do so.

Recall the case of Esther in Chapter 2 who let down her friend as a result of being faced with a choice between letting down her friend and letting down her parents. She decided to let down her friend because she thought that it was the lesser of the two evils. Because Esther held a flexible belief: 'I really don't want to let down people I care about, but sadly I am not immune from doing so and nor do I have to be so immune', she looked at this situation in relative rather than black-and-white terms that helped her to appreciate the complexity of the situation in which she found herself. Thus, she concluded: 'While letting down my friend is wrong, it was the lesser of the two evils and sometimes, as in this case, I can't avoid letting down someone I care about. Life is like that, unfortunately.'

You think you may be penalized rather than receiving retribution

As I have already discussed, when you feel remorse rather than guilt, this is based on the non-extreme belief known as unconditional self-acceptance (USA). Here, you think of yourself as a fallible human being who has done the wrong thing, for example. This involves you rejecting the idea that you are a bad person. When you hold this belief, it encourages you to infer that while you may be penalized for your behaviour, it is unlikely that bad things will happen to you because you deserve retribution for being bad. In short, you believe that because people are fallible rather than bad, they deserve to be penalized rather than punished.

Behaviour that stems from remorse-based rational beliefs

When you hold a set of rational beliefs that lead you to feel remorse but not guilt, you are motivated to face up to breaking your moral/ ethical code, failing to live up to such a code or hurting someone, and to deal with it in the following constructive ways.

You face up to the healthy pain that accompanies the realization that you have 'sinned'

When you hold a set of remorse-based rational beliefs, doing so helps you to face up to the pain that accompanies the realization that you have done something wrong, failed to do the right thing or hurt someone's feelings. Doing so, in turn, helps you to behave in ways that are consistent with the idea that you are prepared to take responsibility for your actions, but in a manner that is based on compassionate self-understanding.

You ask, but do not beg, for forgiveness

When you hold a set of guilt-based irrational beliefs, you tend to beg for forgiveness from the other person that you have wronged, harmed or hurt. However, when you hold an alternative set of rational beliefs, you will ask for such forgiveness when it is appropriate to do so, rather than beg for it. In asking for forgiveness rather than begging for it, you tend to deepen your conviction that you are fallible rather than a bad, despicable creature who can only be raised up if the other person forgives you. Within this framework, if you are not forgiven, you can still forgive yourself for what you did. If you are forgiven, you accept this at face value and do not frequently seek continuing reassurance from the other person that you are forgiven.

You understand the reasons for your wrongdoing and act on your understanding

I have already made the point that guilt is the enemy of understanding. Thus, when you hold a set of guilt-based irrational beliefs, you see the world in black-and-white terms and either deny responsibility for your actions or take all the responsibility and blame yourself. However, in reality, there were probably many influences on your behaviour, with respect both to the situation you were in and to the other people who were involved. Thus, you need to take into account all the variables when striving to understand the complex reasons for your wrongdoing.

Since your remorse-based rational beliefs are flexible and non-extreme they help you to appreciate the complexity of the situation in which you 'sinned' and to act in ways that are consistent with this understanding. This will help you to resist the efforts of others who seek to take advantage of the situation and try to manipulate you through guilt.

You atone for the sin by taking a penalty

When you hold a set of remorse-based rational beliefs and you have done something wrong, failed to do the right thing or hurt someone's feelings, then you take appropriate responsibility for your actions and offer to take a suitable penalty. Such a penalty needs to be differentiated from the punishment, deprivation or penance you tend to accept when you hold a set of guilt-based irrational beliefs, which are likely to be out of proportion to the 'sin' that you committed. The defining characteristic of a suitable penalty is that it is in keeping with what a compassionate understanding person would suggest that you take as a penalty. A punishment, deprivation or penance will tend to be based on what a person lacking in compassion and understanding would suggest that you take. In guilt, such a person is you!

You make appropriate amends

Making amends involves you compensating others who have suffered as a result of your sin. Such compensation may be monetary in nature, but it can also take a less tangible form. A heart-felt apology, together with you outlining what you are going to do to address your future behaviour, can often be a suitable way of making amends to another person. Holding a set of remorse-based rational beliefs helps you to make such appropriate amends.

You do not make excuses for your behaviour or enact other defensive behaviour

As I have said, holding a set of remorse-based rational beliefs leads you to own up to your 'sin' and take an appropriate level of responsibility for it. This, in turn, helps you to refrain from making excuses for your behaviour to involved others or from engaging in other defensive behaviour. This does not mean that you cannot publicly assign responsibility to others who have also contributed, but you acknowledge that when it comes to your own behaviour, the 'buck stops' with you.

You do accept offers of forgiveness

When you feel remorseful about hurting someone, for example, you do not think you are bad. Rather, you take responsibility for your behaviour and accept yourself unconditionally as a fallible human being who has 'sinned'. When the other person offers to forgive you, you will, therefore, tend to accept such an offer, which you are likely to reject when you experience guilt. In the former case, being fallible, you think that you deserve such forgiveness, whereas in the latter case, being bad, you think you are undeserving of it and therefore reject it.

When you routinely and appropriately respond with remorse rather than guilt

When you routinely respond with remorse rather than guilt, then: you experience this emotion only when it is clear that you have broken or failed to live up to your moral code or hurt someone's feelings; you are not easily manipulated by others; you do stand up for yourself; you practise self-care; and you take responsibility for your own feelings and behaviour, but do not think that you are responsible for others' feelings. I now discuss each of these features in turn.

You only feel remorse when it is clear that you have 'sinned'

I pointed out in Chapter 2 that if you are particularly prone to guilt you will think that you often do the wrong thing, fail to do the right thing or hurt the feelings of others. You do this because you hold the following belief, which I called a 'chronic guilt-based general irrational belief':

Whenever I am involved, I must make sure that nothing bad happens or that others' feelings are not hurt. If I don't, and bad things happen and/or others are upset, then it is all my fault and I am a bad person.

However, when your responses are remorse-based rather than guilt-based, then you only think that you have 'sinned' (i.e. done the wrong thing, failed to do the right thing or hurt someone's feelings) when there is clear evidence that you have done so. You are able to do this because you hold the following belief, which I call a 'remorse-based general rational belief':

Whenever I am involved, I want to make sure that nothing bad happens or that others' feelings are not hurt and will do my best in this regard, but I do not have to make sure that this is the case. If I fail in this respect, and bad things happen and/or others are upset, then I will take responsibility for what I am responsible for and will assign responsibility to others when this is indicated. When I have 'sinned', it does not prove that I am a bad person. Rather, I am an unrateable, unique, fallible human being capable of doing good, bad and neutral things.

You then take this belief to relevant situations and are able to look at what happened from a broad perspective, appreciate the complexities involved and only take responsibility for your own actual involvement. When it is clear that you have 'sinned' then you hold a set of specific rational beliefs about this, feel remorseful and take appropriate action.

Let me revisit the case of Josie, who I first discussed in Chapter 2 (see pp. 20–1), and show what difference holding a remorse-based general rational belief would have made to her.

If you recall, Josie had the following chronic guilt-related general irrational belief: 'If I have had dealings with people, I must know that others are not upset in any way as a result. If they are upset, it is my fault and I am a bad person. If I am unsure about how they feel, then I assume that they are upset and I am again the cause, in which case I am a bad person.' She took this belief to a specific situation where her mother asked her over for dinner and Josie said no because she was going out with a friend that night. She explained this to her mother, but was not sure of the latter's reaction. Her chronic guilt-based general irrational belief led her to infer that she had upset her mother. It is as if Josie reasoned: 'Because I can't convince myself that I didn't upset my mother, therefore I did.' Her belief did not allow her to think that her mother was probably accepting of her not going to dinner.

Once Josie had created her inference, she made herself feel guilty about it by holding a specific version of her chronic guilt-based general irrational belief. Thus, 'I upset my mother by turning down her dinner invitation. I absolutely should not have upset my mother in this way and I am a bad person because I did.' Having made herself feel guilty in this way, Josie then thought and acted in ways that were consistent with her guilt-based irrational belief, which had the effect of strengthening this belief.

More generally, Josie experienced guilt whenever others did not show that they were happy in their interactions with her. Her general irrational belief led her (1) to transform her doubt into the inference that she had upset the other person and (2) to think of herself as bad for upsetting them, which she believed she must not do.

In therapy, Josie learned about the dynamics of guilt and was helped by her therapist to develop the following remorse-based general rational belief:

> If I have had dealings with people, I would like to know that others are not upset in any way as a result, but I don't need to know this. If they are upset, I will look at the situation and take responsibility for my contribution, but will also give them responsibility for their contribution. I am not a bad person, if I have done something that contributed to others' hurt feelings. I am a fallible human being who did or said the wrong thing. If I am unsure about how they feel, then I won't assume that they are upset until I find out.

If Josie had taken this belief to the specific situation where her mother asked her over for dinner and Josie said no because she was going out with a friend that night, she would not have assumed that her mother was upset until finding this out. Her belief allowed her to think that her mother was probably accepting of her not going to dinner.

However, if she had discovered that her mother was upset, she would have held a specific version of her remorse-based general irrational belief. Thus, 'I would have preferred not to upset my mother by turning down her dinner invitation, but that does not mean that I must not have done so. I am fallible, not bad, for upsetting my mother in this way.' Having made herself feel remorseful in this way, Josie would then have thought and acted in ways that were consistent with her remorse-based rational belief, which had the effect of strengthening this belief. Thus, she would have seen that her mother was largely responsible for her own upset and, while recognizing that she contributed to this, she would have also acknowledged that she did not cause her mother's upset feelings.

More generally, Josie was able to tolerate her doubt about others' hurt feelings and her role in this. She assumed that others weren't hurt unless she had evidence that they were and accepted herself unconditionally for her contribution to their feelings.

You are not easily manipulated by others

When you routinely respond to 'sinning' with remorse rather than with guilt, others find it much harder to manipulate you than when you have a chronic problem with guilt. While others invite you to think that you have 'sinned' and to define yourself as bad for 'sinning', you do not accept either of these invitations unthinkingly. Rather, you think carefully about the situation and decide for yourself whether you have 'sinned'; if you have, you accept yourself unconditionally for your 'sin', and realize that you are not immune from 'sinning' and nor do you have to be so immune. This independence of thought makes it much harder for you to be manipulated by others' attempts to get you to do something that you don't want to do by inducing your guilt. If you do feel guilty, you realize that you are responsible for making yourself feel this way and that others can't make you feel guilt. This helps you to challenge the irrational beliefs that underpin your guilt and develop remorse-based rational beliefs instead.

You stand up for yourself

If you respond routinely with remorse rather than with guilt to relevant situations, then it is likely that you will stand up for yourself when it is healthy for you to do so. As a result, you tend to have fewer negative events to deal with than people who don't assert themselves. For example, in a work setting you will tend not to get saddled with work that nobody else wants and you won't tend to work longer hours than others. This is because you will say no when people at work try to take advantage of you. You are able to assert yourself even if others may be upset with you because you won't hold yourself responsible for upsetting them, and since you don't believe that you need others' approval, you won't assume that if you stand up for yourself everybody will disapprove of you. You recognize that some might, and if it turns out that they do you will feel sorry about this but will accept yourself unconditionally in the light of such disapproval. However, this will not stop you from standing up for yourself with such people in the future.

You practise self-care

If you routinely respond where appropriate with remorse rather than guilt, then it is likely that you consider both your own interests and those of others, putting your own interests first when it is healthy for you to do so. This is known as self-care. You are able to do this for two reasons. First, you think that, at times, putting your own interests ahead of those of others is healthy and that selflessness, while often praised by others, means that you rarely get what you want in life. You also do not think that putting your interests first means that you are being selfish, since you can see that selfishness means always putting yourself first and being indifferent to others' interests.

You also see that when you practise self-care (sometimes called 'enlightened self-interest'), you sometimes put the interests of others ahead of your own. Self-care is a flexible position, based as it is on a flexible set of beliefs.

You think that while you may contribute to others' upset feelings, you are not responsible for them

Finally, if you routinely respond where appropriate with remorse rather than guilt, then you understand that when you say you have hurt someone's feelings, this is a shorthand way of describing a complex state of affairs rather than a fact. Compare this to chronic guilt, where you do think that you can directly hurt someone's feelings. The complex position is this. When someone has hurt feelings this can be seen as an emotional 'C' in the 'ABC' framework presented in Chapter 1. Your behaviour, from this analysis, is the 'A'. We know, therefore, that the person's upset feelings are largely determined by his or her beliefs about your behaviour and not by your behaviour itself. Before you run away with the idea that this is a psychopath's charter, where you can treat people as badly as you want and they are completely responsible for making themselves feel disturbed about this, this is certainly not the case. When you feel remorse, you take responsibility for your own behaviour and realize that this behaviour contributes to, but does not cause, others' hurt feelings. You therefore are willing to look carefully at your own behaviour (which psychopaths truly do not do) and ask yourself how you could have acted differently so that the other person would have had less reason to disturb him- or herself. Contrast this complex nuanced position to the black-and-white position in chronic guilt, where if someone's feelings are hurt when you are involved, you caused their hurt and are therefore bad – and that is that!

In the following chapter, I will discuss preparing the ground for change. This involves you doing three things: (1) determining whether you have a problem with guilt; if so, (2) determining whether you want to change; and, if you do want to change, (3) accepting yourself for experiencing guilt.

4

Preparing the ground for change

Introduction

So far in the book I have done the following. In Chapter 1, I outlined the 'ABC' model of CBT, and in the following two chapters I used that model to help you understand how CBT conceptualizes guilt (in Chapter 2) and its healthy alternative known as remorse (in Chapter 3). In the following chapters, I am going to show you how you can use CBT to deal with specific guilt problems and with chronic guilt if you suffer from it.

While it would be easy for me to assume that you are reading this book because you recognize that you have a problem with guilt and you want to address this problem, I will refrain from making this assumption, at least until I have dealt with a number of issues that fall under the heading of preparing yourself for change. More specifically I will invite you to do three things in this chapter, in which I discuss preparing the ground for change. First, I am going to invite you to consider whether you have a problem with guilt. If you decide that you do have a problem with this unhealthy negative emotion, I am going to invite you to consider whether you want to address this problem and seek to change it. It is possible that you may acknowledge that you have a problem with guilt and not want to address it. If so, you may read what I have to say about dealing with guilt, but you won't put any of the ideas into practice since you don't have a problem that you want to change. However, before you arrive at this conclusion, please read, with an open mind, what I have to say concerning why people may not want to address their guilt problem. Finally, if you do recognize that you have a guilt problem that you wish to address, I will help you to accept yourself unconditionally for having this problem since, as I will show you, such unconditional self-acceptance encourages change rather than inhibits it.

How to determine whether or not you have a problem with guilt

While I have argued in this book, and especially in Chapter 2, that guilt is an unhealthy negative emotion, it is only when you feel stuck with it or that it is chronic in nature that you are likely to have a problem with it. Even then, you may decide that it is not a problem for you.

However, let me help you decide whether your guilt is problematic in two ways: (1) by looking at specific episodes where you felt guilty and, if necessary, contrasting them with remorse responses, and (2) by considering chronic guilt and again, if necessary, contrasting this with its remorse-based alternative.

Considering specific episodes of guilt and contrasting it, if necessary, with remorse

In Chapters 2 and 3, I discussed CBT's view of guilt (Chapter 2) and remorse (Chapter 3). While doing so I contrasted the thinking and behaviour commonly associated with specific episodes of guilt and that commonly associated with remorse. I summarize this information in Table 4.1 (opposite).

One of the ways, therefore, that you can decide whether or not you have a guilt problem is to take specific examples of this guilt and identify the thinking and behaviour that were associated with your guilt. Use the information in Table 4.1 to help you do this. You do not have to be very precise in identifying your thinking and behavioural responses at this point; a rough idea will suffice.

If it is not clear from doing this that your guilt is problematic, consult Table 4.1 again and this time imagine that you responded with remorse rather than guilt. Then, select from the appropriate sections under 'Remorse' the thinking and behaviour that you would have engaged with if you had experienced that healthy negative emotion. Again, at this stage you do not need to be very precise in your selection. Doing this should help you to see whether your guilt is problematic.

Considering chronic guilt and contrasting it, if necessary, with routinely experienced remorse

If you experience chronic guilt then again you need to determine whether or not this guilt is a problem. I discussed the features of chronic guilt in Chapter 2, but have summarized them in the left-hand column in Table 4.2 (see p. 40).

Table 4.1 Guilt vs remorse

Differences in how you think and behave when you feel guilt or remorse about breaking your moral code, failing to live up to your moral code or hurting others' feelings.

Adversity	• You have broken your moral code. • You have failed to live up to your moral code. • You have hurt someone's feelings.	
Belief	Irrational	Rational
Emotion	**Guilt**	**Remorse**
Behaviour	• You escape from the unhealthy pain of guilt in self-defeating ways. • You beg forgiveness from the person you have wronged. • You promise unrealistically that you will not 'sin' again. • You punish yourself physically or by deprivation. • You defensively disclaim responsibility for wrongdoing. • You reject offers of forgiveness.	• You face up to the healthy pain that accompanies the realization that you have 'sinned'. • You ask, but do not beg, for forgiveness. • You understand the reasons for your wrongdoing and act on your understanding. • You atone for the 'sin' by taking a penalty. • You make appropriate amends. • You do not make excuses for your behaviour or enact other defensive behaviour. • You do accept offers of forgiveness.
Thinking	• You conclude that you have definitely committed the 'sin'. • You assume more personal responsibility than the situation warrants. • You assign far less responsibility to others than is warranted. • You dismiss possible mitigating factors for your behaviour. • You only see your behaviour in a guilt-related context and fail to put it into an overall context. • You think that you will receive retribution.	• You take into account all relevant data when judging whether or not you have 'sinned'. • You assume an appropriate level of personal responsibility. • You assign an appropriate level of responsibility to others. • You take into account mitigating factors. • You put your behaviour into an overall context. • You think you may be penalized rather than receive retribution.

Table 4.2 The different consequences of chronic guilt and routinely and appropriately experienced remorse

Chronic guilt	When you routinely and appropriately respond with remorse rather than guilt
• You feel guilty much of the time.	• You only feel remorse when it is clear that you have 'sinned'.
• You are easily manipulated by others.	• You are not easily manipulated by others.
• You fail to stand up for yourself.	• You stand up for yourself.
• You fail to practise self-care.	• You practise self-care.
• You think that you are responsible for others' upset feelings.	• You think that while you may contribute to others' upset feelings, you are not responsible for them.

Identify the features of your own chronic guilt from this list and then determine whether or not you consider your chronic guilt a problem. If you are still undecided consult the right-hand column of Table 4.2 and identify the remorse-based alternatives to the features of your chronic guilt. This should help you to see that your chronic guilt is a problem for you.

Deciding whether you want to address your guilt problem

Once you have concluded that you have a guilt problem then you need to decide whether you want to address it and seek to develop a healthier way of dealing with times when you have, or think you have, broken your moral code, failed to live up to your moral code or hurt someone's feelings. To help you to make your decision, I have provided information concerning what it would be like to experience remorse as an alternative to guilt both at a specific episodic level and at a more general level (see Tables 4.1 and 4.2).

If you are still unclear about whether or not you want to address your guilt problem, I suggest that you carry out a cost–benefit analysis (CBA) on your guilt problem and remorse-based alternative. This is how you carry out such a cost–benefit analysis.

The CBA form found in Figure 4.1 is an example to help you. Copy it out, leaving plenty of space for each section. It is a good idea to use separate pages for the problem, the alternative and your responses to the advantages and disadvantages.

The problem: [write the problem here]

Advantages of the problem

Short-term advantages

For myself

For others

Long-term advantages

For myself

For others

Disadvantages of the problem

Short-term disadvantages

For myself

For others

Long-term disadvantages

For myself

For others

The alternative: [write the alternative here]

Advantages of the alternative

Short-term advantages

For myself

For others

Long-term advantages

For myself

For others

Disadvantages of the alternative

Short-term disadvantages

For myself

For others

Long-term disadvantages

For myself

For others

Figure 4.1 An example of a cost–benefit analysis form

Here are a set of instructions to help you complete your CBA form:

At the top of the first page state the problem as you see it.

Then state the advantages you think you get from having the problem. As you can see, such advantages may be (1) short-term and/or long-term and (2) for yourself and/or for others.

Next, state the disadvantages you think you get from having the problem. As you can see, such disadvantages may again be (1) short-term and/or long-term and (2) for yourself and/or for others.

At the top of the second page state the alternative to the problem as you see it.

Then state the advantages you think you will get from developing the alternative to the problem. As you can see, such advantages may be (1) short-term and/or long-term and (2) for yourself and/or for others.

Next, state the disadvantages you think you will get from developing the alternative to the problem. As you can see, such disadvantages may again be (1) short-term and/or long-term and (2) for yourself and/or for others.

Stand back and on a separate piece of paper write down responses to any advantages of having the problem that you have stated and to any disadvantages of developing the alternative to the problem that you have mentioned. It may help you to do this if you imagine that you are helping your best friend to counter both the advantages of the same problem and the disadvantages of the same alternative.

You should now be in a position to commit yourself to addressing your guilt problem and have some idea of what your goal is with respect to this problem, although you will have a chance later to be more specific about goal-setting.

The case of Eric

Eric recognized that he had a problem with guilt about upsetting his parents whenever he put himself first over their own interests. However, he was unsure whether he wanted to address this problem so he decided to do a cost–benefit analysis about feeling guilt for hurting his parents' feelings versus feeling remorse for hurting their feelings. Then he stood back and considered the advantages of feeling guilty and the disadvantages of feeling remorse. Figure 4.2 on pages 44–5 shows how he responded to these advantages and disadvantages.

Responding to the advantages of feeling guilty

In this section, Eric shows how he responded to the advantages of his problem.

Responding to the short-term advantages of feeling guilt
For myself,

Advantage: 'Guilt shows that I care about my parents' feelings.'
Response: 'Guilt may show that I care about my parents' feelings, but it also shows that I feel disturbed about upsetting them. Remorse, on the other hand, shows that I care about their feelings without disturbing myself when I upset them.'

Advantage: 'Guilt is proof that I am taking the issue seriously.'
Response: 'Guilt may be proof that I am taking the issue of hurting my parents' feelings seriously, but it comes at a price: disturbance, and me not looking after my own interests at all. Remorse shows that I am taking the issue seriously, but without disturbance and self-denial.'

Responding to the long-term advantages of feeling guilt
For myself,

Advantage: 'I get the satisfaction of putting my parents first in the same way as they put me first when I was a child.'
Response: 'While my parents often put me first as a child, they also went out and got a babysitter for me. So I can also find a balance between putting myself first and putting them first. Also, even if I do want to put them first all the time, I can do this by choice rather than because I would feel guilty if I didn't.'

Responding to the short-term advantages of feeling guilt
For others,

Advantage: 'My parents get what they want in the short term.'
Response: 'They may get what they want, but it wouldn't be that bad if they learned that, even as they enter their twilight years, some of the time it's all right for me to look after my own interests.'

Advantage: 'My parents don't think I am selfish when I do what they want.'
Response: 'If my parents thought I was selfish, that would be painful for them. However, it would not be true that I am selfish and I have to weigh up putting myself first some of the time, and risk the fact that they might find that painful, versus me choosing to put them first all the time and therefore sparing them pain. I am going to choose the former, but will be remorseful about my parents being in pain because I don't want that. I am choosing the former because it is fairer to all involved.'

The problem: Guilt about hurting my parents' feelings

Advantages of the problem (i.e. guilt about hurting my parents' feelings)

Short-term advantages

For myself
1 It shows that I care about my parents' feelings.
2 It is proof that I am taking the issue seriously.

For others
1 My parents get what they want in the short term.
2 My parents don't think I am selfish when I do what they want.

Long-term advantages

For myself
1 I get the satisfaction of putting parents first in the same way as they put me first when I was a child.

For others
1 By putting my parents first, they have an easier life, which they deserve.

Disadvantages of the problem (i.e. guilt about hurting my parents' feelings)

Short-term disadvantages

For myself
1 I feel disturbed in the short term when I hurt my parents' feelings.
2 By not putting myself first at all I feel disturbed in the short term.

For others
1 My parents feel upset in the short term when I put myself first.
2 My parents don't get to do what they want in the short term.

Long-term disadvantages

For myself
1 I feel disturbed in the long term when I hurt my parents' feelings.
2 By not putting myself first at all I feel disturbed in the long term.

For others
1 My parents feel upset in the long term when I put myself first.
2 My parents don't get to do what they want in the long term.

Figure 4.2 Eric's cost–benefit analysis form

Responding to the long-term advantages of feeling guilt
For others,

> *Advantage*: 'By putting my parents first, they have an easier life, which they deserve.'
> *Response*: 'While I can decide to put my parents first all the time and give them an easier life, I am choosing a way forward so that we all get some of what we want. While my parents may suffer to some degree as a result, this is the unfortunate consequence of my decision. I can make this decision because guilt is not driving it. When guilt drives my decision I put them first all the time, which leads me to experience all the suffering. This is not fair and I don't want to continue to go down this route.'

The alternative: Remorse about hurting my parents' feelings

Advantages of the alternative (i.e. remorse about hurting my parents' feelings)

Short-term advantages	Long-term advantages
For myself	*For myself*
1 I get to do some of what I want as well as putting my parents' interests first some of the time.	1 I get to do some of what I want as well as putting my parents' interests first some of the time.
2 When my parents do show they are upset I don't feel disturbed in the short term.	2 When my parents do show they are upset I don't feel disturbed in the long term.
3 In the short term it shows that I care without feeling disturbed when my parents are upset.	3 In the long term it shows that I care without feeling disturbed when my parents are upset.
For others	*For others*
1 My parents would be pleased that I don't feel disturbed in the short term.	1 My parents would be pleased that I don't feel disturbed in the long term.

Disadvantages of the alternative (i.e. remorse about hurting my parents' feelings)

Short-term disadvantages	Long-term disadvantages
For myself	*For myself*
None.	None.
For others	*For others*
1 My parents feel upset when I don't put them first.	1 My parents will feel more upset than they would if I felt guilt.
2 On a specific occasion my parents don't get to do what they want.	2 My parents don't get to do what they want as much as they would if I felt guilt.

Responding to the disadvantages of feeling remorse

In this section, Eric shows how he responded to the disadvantages of his alternative.

Responding to the short-term disadvantages of feeling remorse

For others,

> *Disadvantage*: 'My parents feel upset when I don't put them first.'
> *Response*: 'That is true, but that is not a reason for me not to put myself first some of the time. I am trying to ensure that we all get what we want some of the time.'
> *Disadvantage*: 'On a specific occasion my parents don't get to do what they want.'

Response: 'That is also true, but once again that is not a reason for me not to put myself first some of the time. I am trying to ensure that there is balance in our relationship.'

Responding to the long-term disadvantages of feeling remorse
For others,

Disadvantage: 'My parents will feel more upset than they would if I felt guilt.'
Response: 'That is because if I felt guilt I would put them first all the time and myself first none of the time. I am sorry if they feel upset, but I am trying to have a balanced relationship with them.'

Disadvantage: 'My parents don't get to do what they want as much as they would if I felt guilt.'
Response: 'Again true, but then I don't get to do anything I want to do if I put them first all the time. That is unfair to me and I am not going to do that any more!'

Eric's conclusion
After Eric had carried out a cost–benefit analysis on his guilt about hurting his parents' feelings and the alternative to this problem, and he had responded to the advantages of his problem and to the disadvantages of the alternative, Eric decided that he definitely wanted to address his guilt problem.

Accept yourself unconditionally for having a guilt problem

You have now identified that you have a problem with guilt and have decided to address it. Before you take steps to bring about change, it is useful to consider whether you are depreciating yourself for having a guilt problem. If you are, it is important that you first work to accept yourself unconditionally for having this problem before you tackle it. Why? Because if you depreciate yourself for having a guilt problem (including the behavioural and thinking components of this problem), you give yourself two problems for the price of one – your guilt problem and the emotional problem that you have about your guilt problem. This latter problem is known as a meta-emotional problem (literally, an emotional problem about an emotional problem). When you have a meta-emotional problem about your guilt problem, it is like trying to climb up a hill with a ball and chain around your leg. It hampers your progress. Therefore, if you do have a meta-emotional problem about your guilt problem it is important that you address it before tackling your guilt problem.

The most prevalent meta-emotional problem that people have about their guilt problem is based on a self-depreciation belief. Thus, you may feel ashamed of having a guilt problem because you think it proves that you are defective; you may feel unhealthily angry with yourself because you think that you are an idiot for failing to assert yourself, or you feel depressed because you think that putting others first reconfirms that you are worthless.

Therefore, if you depreciate yourself for having a guilt problem, it is important that you work to accept yourself unconditionally instead. You can do this by working to believe the following:

- While your guilt problem may be bad, this is just a part of you and cannot define you.
- You are fallible, which means that you have what Dr Maxie C. Maultsby Jr once called an 'incurable error-making tendency', and therefore your guilt problem is evidence of your fallibility rather than your worthlessness.
- If you have worth as a human being it is because you are alive, fallible, too complex to be rated, unique and in flux. All these are features that do not change as long as you exist. Thus, your worth as a human being does not change whether or not you have a guilt problem.

You do not have to accept yourself fully for having a guilt problem before you tackle it. However, it is important that you make some progress on this issue and that you respond to any self-depreciating thoughts about having a guilt problem when you become aware of them.

You have now prepared the ground for change. In the following chapter, I am going to show you how you can define your guilt problem and set a goal with respect to this defined problem.

5

Defining your guilt problem and setting a goal with respect to this defined problem

Introduction

You have prepared the ground for change and are ready to begin to tackle your guilt problem. If you have a specific guilt problem then the first step that you need to take is to define this problem. If you have a chronic guilt problem, it is likely that you have a problem with guilt in quite a number of areas. Despite this, it is useful to take one specific guilt problem and deal with this first, before tackling the chronic nature of your guilt. I will show you how you can deal with chronic guilt in Chapter 10. In this chapter, however, I am going to help you to define your guilt problem and to set a realistic goal with respect to this problem.

Define your guilt problem: general issues

The first step is for you to define your guilt problem in your own words. However, it is useful for you to include the following points when you do so.

The context of your guilt problem

You experience your guilt problem within a context and it is useful for you to include this context in your description of your guilt problem.

Your emotion

Your emotion is, of course, guilt and this is the emotional 'C' in the 'ABC' framework. If you are still unsure whether your problematic emotion is guilt rather than remorse, consult Table 4.1 in Chapter 4 (see p. 39).

What you are most guilty about

You will know by now that you feel guilty about:

* breaking your moral or ethical code;

- failing to live up to your moral or ethical code;
- hurting someone.

You feel guilty about these inferences at 'A' in the 'ABC' framework whether they are true or not. At this point it is useful to provide content to these inferences so that you are clear about what moral or ethical code(s) you have broken and who you have hurt.

Your behaviour

When you experience your guilt problem you will have a tendency to act in certain ways. These will be an elaboration of your guilt or will be an attempt to get rid of this feeling. Such behaviour is the behavioural 'C' in the 'ABC' framework.

Define your guilt problem: applying the general issues

Let me now show you how you can apply this to guilt about (1) breaking your moral/ethical code, (2) failing to live up to your moral/ethical code or (3) hurting others.

When your guilt problem involves acts of commission

When you feel guilty about doing things that break your moral or ethical code, I suggest that you include some or all of the following in your description.

The context

Here, I suggest you look for patterns in the situations in which you experience your guilt about acts of commission. This is the context of your guilt problem.

Your emotion (emotional 'C')

This will be guilt.

What you are guilty about ('A')

Specify the content theme of your moral/ethical code violation.

What you did when you felt guilty (behavioural 'C')

When you feel guilty about acts of commission, your guilt-related irrational beliefs have been activated and these will influence your subsequent behaviour. In your description of your guilt problem list the major way in which you behave. This may either elaborate your guilt or be designed to avoid it or cut it short.

Teresa's description of her guilt problem about acts of commission

Here is Teresa's description of her guilt problem which features moral code violation.

> Whenever I see people smoke, I feel an urge to smoke myself. If I have an opportunity to smoke I take it even though I am trying to give up. When I do so I feel guilty about breaking my promise to my daughter that I would stop smoking and end up by engaging in other self-defeating activity to stop me feeling guilty.

You will note that Teresa's description contains the following:

> Context = 'Whenever I see people smoke, I feel an urge to smoke myself. If I have an opportunity to smoke I take it even though I am trying to give up.'
> Emotion at 'C' = Guilt.
> Moral/ethical code violation at 'A' = 'Breaking my promise to my daughter that I would stop smoking.'
> Behaviour at 'C' = Engaging in other self-defeating activity.

When your guilt problem involves acts of omission

When you feel guilty about not doing things that are in line with your moral or ethical code, I suggest that you include some or all of the following in your description.

The context

Here, I suggest you look for patterns in the situations in which you experience your guilt about acts of omission. This is the context of your guilt problem.

Your emotion (emotional 'C')

This will be guilt.

What you are guilty about ('A')

Specify the content theme of your failure to live up to your moral/ethical code.

What you did when you felt guilty (behavioural 'C')

When you feel guilty about acts of omission, your guilt-related irrational beliefs have been activated and these will influence your subsequent behaviour. In your description of your guilt problem, list the major way in which you behave. Again, this may either elaborate your guilt or be designed to avoid it or cut it short.

Bernice's description of her guilt problem about acts of omission

Here is Bernice's description of her guilt problem, which features failure to live up to her moral code.

> Whenever I see people in trouble, I want to go to their aid, but I am afraid to do so. When I fail to help others, I feel guilty about failing to live up to my moral code, and to punish myself I harm myself in some way.

You will note that Bernice's example contains the following:

> Context = 'Whenever I see people in trouble, I want to go to their aid, but I am afraid to do so.'
> Emotion at 'C' = Guilt.
> Moral/ethical code violation at 'A' = Failing to help people in need.
> Behaviour at 'C' = 'I harm myself.'

When your guilt problem involves hurting others

When you feel guilty about hurting others' feelings, I suggest that you include some or all of the following in your description.

The context

Here, I suggest you look for patterns in the situations in which you experience your guilt about hurting others. This is the context of your guilt problem.

Your emotion (emotional 'C')

This will be guilt.

What you are guilty about ('A')

Specify the theme involved in hurting others.

What you did when you felt guilty (behavioural 'C')

When you feel guilty about hurting others, your guilt-related irrational beliefs have been activated and again these will influence your subsequent behaviour. In your description of your guilt problem, list the major way in which you behave. As before, this may either elaborate your guilt or be designed to avoid it or cut it short.

Eric's description of his guilt problem about hurting others

> Whenever I want to put my own interests ahead of those of my parents, they feel upset and I feel guilty about hurting their

feelings. The consequence of this is that I put their interests before my own and don't do what I want to do.

You will note that Eric's description contains the following:

Context = 'A wish to put my interests first.'
Emotion at 'C' = Guilt.
Theme of hurting others at 'A' = 'Hurting my parents' feelings.'
Behaviour at 'C' = 'Putting my parents' interests ahead of my own.'

Set a realistic goal with respect to your guilt problem: general issues

In setting a realistic goal with respect to your guilt problem, it is important that you do so in your own words. However, it is useful for you to include the following points when you do so.

The context

The context in which you experience your guilt problem and what this problem is about are the same in your problem and when you set a goal.

When you experience your guilt problem it is within a context and about an 'A' (i.e. breaking a moral/ethical code, failing to live up your moral/ethical code or hurting others). Thus, when you set a goal with respect to your problem, the context and the 'A' will be the same but your responses (emotional and behavioural) will be different.

Your emotional goal

Since your emotional problem is guilt, you need to set an emotional goal which is a healthier response to your 'A' and the context in which you experienced it. In CBT the healthy negative emotional alternative to guilt is remorse (see Table 4.1 in Chapter 4, p. 39) and therefore you should consider this as your emotional goal when you break your moral/ethical code, fail to live up your moral/ethical code or hurt others. Since the 'A' is negative, your emotional goal also needs to be negative (after all, it is unhealthy to feel positive or neutral about a negative event), but it also needs to be healthier than guilt. Remorse fits the bill on both counts and is the emotional 'C' in the 'ABC' framework outlining your goal.

Your behavioural goal

When you experience remorse, your behaviour will be more constructive than the behaviour associated with guilt. This constructive behaviour will be your behavioural goal and is the behavioural 'C' in the 'ABC' framework, outlining your goal.

Set a realistic goal with respect to your guilt problem: applying the general issues

Let me now show you how you can apply this to setting your goal with respect to your guilt problem about (1) breaking your moral/ethical code, (2) failing to live up to your moral/ethical code or (3) hurting others.

Setting your goal when your guilt problem involves acts of commission

In setting your goal about doing things that break your moral or ethical code, remember that your context and your 'A' will be the same as in your guilt problem.

The context

This will be the same as in your guilt problem about acts of commission.

Your emotional goal (new emotional 'C')

This will be remorse.

What you are remorseful about ('A')

This will be same as in your guilt problem about acts of commission.

What you can do when you feel remorseful (new behavioural 'C')

This behaviour will be a constructive behavioural alternative to the behaviour you carried out in your guilt problem.

Teresa's goal

Here is Teresa's description of her goal with respect to her guilt problem about her moral code violation.

> Whenever I see people smoke, I feel an urge to smoke myself. If I have an opportunity to smoke I take it even though I am trying to give up. When I do so I want to feel remorseful rather than guilty about breaking my promise to my daughter that I would stop smoking. I want to engage in activities designed to help me deal with my urges rather than engaging in other self-defeating activity to stop me feeling guilty.

You will note that Teresa's goal contains the following:

Context = 'Whenever I see people smoke, I feel an urge to smoke myself. If I have an opportunity to smoke I take it even though I am trying to give up.' This is the same context as in her guilt problem.

Emotional goal at 'C' = Remorse.

Moral/ethical code violation at 'A' = 'Breaking my promise to my daughter that I would stop smoking.' This is the same 'A' as in her guilt problem.

Behavioural goal at 'C' = 'Engaging in activities designed to help me deal with my urges rather than engaging in other self-defeating activity to stop me feeling guilty.'

Setting your goal when your guilt problem involves acts of omission

In setting your goal about failing to do things that are consistent with your moral or ethical code, remember that your context and your 'A' will be the same as in your guilt problem.

The context

This will be the same as in your guilt problem about acts of omission.

Your emotional goal (new emotional 'C')

This will be remorse.

What you feel remorseful about ('A')

This will be the same as in your guilt problem about acts of omission.

What you can do when you feel remorseful (new behavioural 'C')

This behaviour will be a constructive alternative to the behaviour you carried out in your guilt problem.

Bernice's goal

Here is Bernice's goal with respect to her guilt problem about failing to live up to her moral code.

Whenever I see people in trouble, I want to go to their aid, but I am afraid to do so. When I fail to help others, I want to feel remorseful rather guilty about failing to live up to my moral code and to learn how to overcome my fear about helping others in trouble rather than harm myself in some way.

You will note that Bernice's goal contains the following:

Context = 'Whenever I see people in trouble, I want to go to their aid, but I am afraid to do so.' This is the same context as in her guilt problem.
Emotional goal at 'C' = Remorse.
Moral/ethical code violation at 'A' = 'I fail to help people in need.' This is the same 'A' as in her guilt problem.
Behavioural goal at 'C' = 'To learn to deal with my anxiety about helping others in trouble rather than harm myself in some way.'

Setting your goal when your guilt problem involves hurting others

In setting your goal about hurting others, remember that your context and your 'A' will be the same as in your guilt problem.

The context

This will be the same as in your guilt problem about hurting others.

Your emotional goal (new emotional 'C')

This will be remorse.

What you are remorseful about ('A')

This will be the same as in your guilt problem about hurting others.

What you can do when you feel remorseful (new behavioural 'C')

This behaviour will be a constructive alternative to the behaviour you carried out in your guilt problem.

Eric's goal

Here is Eric's goal with respect to his guilt problem about hurting others.

Whenever I want to put my own interests ahead of those of my parents, they feel upset. I want to feel remorseful rather than guilty about hurting their feelings. I want to put my interests before their interests and do what I want to do rather than putting their interests before mine.

You will note that Eric's goal contains the following:

Context = 'A wish to put my interests first.'
Emotional goal at 'C' = Remorse.
Theme of hurting others at 'A' = 'Hurting my parents' feelings.'

This is the same as in his guilt problem about hurting others. Behavioural goal at 'C' = 'I want to put my interests before their interests and do what I want to do rather than putting their interests first.'

In the next chapter, I will show you how to assess a specific example of your guilt problem, as you need to know what to address so that you can achieve your goal.

6

Assessing a specific example of your guilt problem and setting goals with respect to this specific example

Introduction

Once you have defined your guilt problem and set a goal with respect to this problem, you are ready to assess the problem. Assessment is important because it helps to pinpoint the factors that you need to address and change in order to achieve your goal. I also suggest that you set goals with respect to this assessment. This again gives you a clear idea of what you are aiming to achieve in related future episodes.

Selecting a concrete example of your guilt problem to assess

In my opinion, at the outset it is best for you to assess a concrete example of your guilt problem. Doing so will provide you with the specific information that will facilitate an accurate assessment of the concrete example that will, in turn, assist you in dealing effectively with the factors that account for your guilt.

When thinking of selecting a concrete example of your guilt problem, you might choose:

- a vivid example of the problem
- a recent example of the problem
- a typical example of the problem
- a future example of the problem.

If relevant, I recommend selecting a future example of the problem because it gives you an opportunity to practise thinking and acting in different ways in an up-and-coming situation. With past examples you can only practise thinking and acting differently retrospectively.

You will be assessing the following elements:

1 the situation you were in when you felt (or predicted that you would feel) guilty;

2 the behavioural and thinking components of your guilt response ('C');
3 what you felt (or predicted that you would feel) most guilty about ('A');
4 the irrational beliefs that underpinned (or would underpin) your guilt ('B').

You will also be setting goals with respect to the second and fourth of these elements.

Describe the situation

When assessing a concrete example of your guilt example, it is important to locate that example within a specific situation which you should describe. In your description, include only what a video camera with an audio channel would record. Thus, try not to make any inferences about what happened. An inference is a hunch about what happened that goes beyond the data at hand.

It is easier to describe something that has happened rather than something that may happen in the future since, by definition, a future prediction is inferential. However, it can be done: let me demonstrate this by referring to the case of Eric, who we first met in Chapter 4.

Eric's description of the situation

Eric's description of the situation in his chosen concrete example of his guilt problem was as follows:

Tomorrow, I want to tell my parents that I won't be able to see them this weekend. My mother will cry and my father will tell me that I am selfish.

Although this is a future situation, Eric predicts events that would be picked up audio-visually if they occurred. A camera would capture his mother crying and an audio channel would pick up his father saying: 'You are selfish.'

Compare this with a statement that Eric could have made. The inferences that he makes are in italics:

Tomorrow, I want to tell my parents that I won't be able to see them this weekend. In doing so, *I will hurt my mother* and *infuriate my father*, who *will accuse me* of being selfish.

Note the following about Eric's second statement. The phrases 'I will hurt my mother' and 'infuriate my father' are inferential in two ways. First, they posit a causal relationship which goes beyond mere description. Second, the terms 'hurt' and 'infuriate' are also inferences about the inner states of his mother and father respectively. Contrast this with Eric's statement where he predicted that his mother would cry and that his father would tell him that he (Eric) was selfish. These are observable events.

The statement 'my father will accuse me' is also inferential since while a video camera with an audio channel would pick up the words 'You are selfish', they would not pick up an 'accusation'.

I want to reiterate that an inference may well be correct. Thus, it may be the case that Eric's mother felt hurt and his father felt infuriated, but it is also feasible that they may have been feigning these emotions. The point is that at this opening stage of the assessment process it is useful to describe the situation.

Remember Cluedo

When describing the situation you were in or may face when experiencing your guilt problem, it is useful to remember the rules of Cluedo, the board game. The goal of this game is to discover the name of the murderer, where the murder took place and the implement with which it was committed. This 'who–what–where' approach is a good guide to the specificity that you need to aim for when describing the situation. To reiterate a point I made above, refrain from including inferences of the description of the situation.

Assess 'C'

After describing the situation that you were in (or predict that you will be in), I recommend that you begin by assessing 'C' rather than 'A' since, in my experience, it is easier to identify 'A' when you have already identified 'C' than without this information. However, you may assess 'A' before 'C' if you wish.

Identify the three components of your guilt response

When you come to assess 'C', I suggest that you first identify the elements of your guilt response and then what would constitute the three elements of a healthier response.

You will recall from Chapter 1 that there are three components of what might be called your guilt response in your chosen concrete example: the emotional component, the behavioural component and the thinking component. It is important to assess each component.

Identify the emotional component

The emotional component here is, of course, guilt.

Identify the behavioural component

The behavioural component concerns overt behaviour or action tendencies that you engage in or 'feel like' engaging in when you feel guilty. The following are the most common behaviours associated with guilt.

> You escape from the unhealthy pain of guilt in self-defeating ways.
> You beg forgiveness from the person you have wronged.
> You promise unrealistically that you will not 'sin' again.
> You punish yourself physically or by deprivation.
> You defensively disclaim responsibility for wrongdoing.
> You reject offers of forgiveness.

Use this as a guide to select how you acted in the specific situation in which you felt guilty.

Eric's behaviour   Because he was feeling guilty, Eric decided not to tell his parents that he wanted time for himself over the weekend and instead he put their interests first.

Identify the thinking component

The thinking component associated with guilt appears below. As you can see, these thoughts are highly distorted and skewed to the negative. They may be in words or in mental pictures. Use this list as a guide to select how you thought in the specific situation in which you felt guilty.

> You conclude that you have definitely committed the sin.
> You assume more personal responsibility than the situation warrants.
> You assign far less responsibility to others than is warranted.
> You dismiss possible mitigating factors for your behaviour.
> You only see your behaviour in a guilt-related context and fail to put it into an overall context.
> You think that you will receive retribution.

Eric's thinking   When he felt guilty, Eric thought that if he did put himself first, not only would he hurt his parents but he would also be punished in some way.

Set goals with respect to each of the three components

You need to set goals so that you know what you are striving for when you deal effectively with guilt in a concrete situation. The three components of your goal are as follows:

Set your emotional goal

Your emotional goal is remorse rather than guilt (or whatever synonym you prefer for the term 'remorse'). Remorse is a healthy negative emotion which is an appropriate response to doing the wrong thing, not doing the right thing or hurting someone's feelings. It helps you to think objectively about the situation and your response to it and helps you to move on with your life rather than get stuck or bogged down.

Set your behavioural goal

Your behavioural goal should reflect actions that are based on remorse about doing the wrong thing, not doing the right thing or hurting someone's feelings, rather than on guilt. The following are the most common behaviours associated with remorse.

You face up to the healthy pain that accompanies the realization that you have 'sinned'.

You ask, but do not beg, for forgiveness.

You understand the reasons for your wrongdoing and act on your understanding.

You atone for the 'sin' by taking a penalty.

You make appropriate amends.

You do not make excuses for your behaviour or enact other defensive behaviour.

You do accept offers of forgiveness.

You may wish to compare these behaviours with those associated with guilt that I presented on p. 60.

Eric's behavioural goal   Eric decided that he would tell his parents that he wanted time for himself over the weekend and would not put their interests first.

Set your thinking goal

As well as setting behavioural goals related to the feeling of remorse about doing the wrong thing, not doing the right thing or hurting someone's feelings, it is also important that you set thinking goals associated with this emotion. The following are the most common forms of thinking associated with remorse rather than guilt. They are balanced and realistic. Again, you may wish to compare these forms of thinking with those associated with guilt that I presented on p. 60.

> You take into account all relevant data when judging whether or not you have 'sinned'.
> You assume an appropriate level of personal responsibility.
> You assign an appropriate level of responsibility to others.
> You take into account mitigating factors.
> You put your behaviour into overall context.
> You think you may be penalized rather than receive retribution.

As the above list shows, the dominant feature of thinking associated with remorse is that it is realistic and balanced. Again, please remember that such thinking may be in words or in mental pictures.

Eric's thinking goal   Eric's thinking goal was to think that it was unlikely that he would be punished for putting himself first even though his parents would be hurt.

Assess 'A'

Once you are clear about your guilt response at 'C', you are ready to discover what you are guilty about in the concrete example you have chosen. You will know by now that your experience of guilt is likely to be about one of the following general categories:

- breaking your moral or ethical code
- failing to live up to your moral or ethical code
- hurting others.

I suggest that you select the category that best describes what you are guilty about in general terms. Then make the category as specific as you can. Thus:

- If you felt, or think that you will feel, guilty about breaking your moral or ethical code, be specific about what you did and about the moral/ethical code that you broke.

- If you felt, or think that you will feel, guilty about failing to live up to your moral or ethical code, be specific about what you failed to do and the moral/ethical code that you did not live up to.
- If you felt, or think that you will feel, guilty about hurting others, be specific about who these others are, what you did (or will do) to hurt them and the nature of their hurt.

Assume temporarily that 'A' is true

The CBT model of guilt is based on the idea that your guilt is largely determined not by breaking your moral/ethical code, failing to live up to this code or hurting others at 'A', but by the beliefs that you hold at 'B' about 'A'. Thus, you need to identify these beliefs. However, in order to do so, you need to assume temporarily that 'A' is (or will be) true. Thus, you need to assume that (1) you have broken, or will break, your moral/ethical code as specified above, (2) you have failed, or will fail, to live up to your moral/ethical code as specified above or (3) you have, or will, hurt others as specified above.

If you don't assume that 'A' is true, you may be tempted to persuade yourself that 'A' is false. If you manage to do so, this will help you feel better in the very short term but will do nothing to help you to address the main sources of your guilt response, which are the specific irrational beliefs that you held about your specific 'A' as specified above.

Eric's 'A'

Eric considered that he would feel guilty about hurting his mother's feelings and infuriating his father if he told them that he could not see them over the weekend. He assumed that this 'A' was true.

Identify your specific irrational beliefs and alternative specific rational beliefs

In CBT, guilt is understood to largely stem from the irrational beliefs that you hold about breaking your moral/ethical code, failing to live up to this code or hurting others. Additionally, remorse (the healthy alternative to guilt) is understood to largely stem from the rational beliefs that you hold about these three inference themes.

Identify the specific irrational beliefs that underpin your guilt

As I discussed in Chapter 2, the main irrational beliefs that underpin guilt are rigid beliefs and self-depreciation beliefs. Since you are assessing a concrete example of your guilt, your task at this point is to identify the specific irrational beliefs (rigid and self-depreciation beliefs) that underpin your specific guilt response in the concrete situation that you have chosen to assess.

Eric's specific guilt-related irrational beliefs

Eric identified the following rigid and self-depreciation beliefs that underpinned his guilt response in his concrete example.

> *Rigid belief*: 'I must not hurt my mother and infuriate my father.'
> *Self-depreciation belief*: 'I would be a bad person if I were to do so.'

Identify the specific rational beliefs that would underpin your remorse

As I discussed in Chapter 2, the main rational beliefs that underpin remorse are flexible beliefs and unconditional self-acceptance (USA) beliefs. Your task at this point is to identify the specific rational beliefs (flexible and USA beliefs) that would underpin your specific remorse response in the concrete situation that you have chosen to assess. Remember that the remorse response is your goal in dealing with this concrete situation.

Eric's specific remorse-related rational beliefs

Eric identified the following flexible and unconditional self-acceptance beliefs that would underpin his remorse response should he hurt his mother's feelings and infuriate his father in the concrete situation that he was focusing on.

> *Flexible belief*: 'I don't want to hurt my mother and infuriate my father, but sadly it does not follow that I must not do so.'
> *Unconditional self-acceptance belief*: 'I would not be a bad person if I were to hurt my mother and infuriate my father. I would be a fallible human being who would be doing something that I do not want to do in order to do something that would be in my healthy interests.'

Having formulated your specific irrational and rational beliefs, the next step is for you to question them. I will show you how to do this in the following chapter.

7

Questioning your beliefs

Introduction

You have now assessed a concrete example of your guilt problem. The last factor you identified was the specific irrational beliefs that underpinned your guilt response and the specific alternative rational beliefs that would underpin your remorse response, which is what you are aiming for. The next step is for you to question these beliefs, the purpose of which is for you to see clearly why your irrational beliefs are irrational and why your alternative rational beliefs are rational. When you have done this you are more likely to commit yourself to weakening your conviction in the former and strengthening your conviction in the latter.

Prepare yourself for the belief-questioning process

Before you embark on this questioning process you need to make sure that you fully understand and agree with two connections that you have made in the assessment process.

Understand and agree with the 'iB–guilt' and 'rB–remorse' connections

It is very important that you understand and agree with the connection between your irrational beliefs and your feelings of guilt at 'C' – known as the *'iB–guilt' connection*. It is also important that you understand the connection between your rational beliefs and the alternative healthy negative emotion to guilt which, as discussed in this book, is remorse. This is known as the *'rB–remorse' connection*. This is how you can make these two connections.

> Ask yourself: 'Can I see that as long as I believe . . . (state 'iBs'), then I will feel guilt? On the other hand, can I see that if I believe . . . (state 'rBs'), then I will feel remorse?'

Eric's example

Can I see that as long as I believe 'I must not hurt my mother and infuriate my father and I would be a bad person if I were to do so', then I will feel guilty?

On the other hand, can I see that I will feel remorse if I believe 'I don't want to hurt my mother and infuriate my father, but sadly it does not follow that I must not do so. I would not be a bad person if I were to do so. I would be a fallible human being who did something that I did not want to do in order to do something that was in my healthy interests'?

You need to understand these two connections before engaging in the belief-questioning process to be described in the sections that follow. If you are having difficulty doing so, review the material in Chapters 1, 2 and 3.

Dealing with your doubts about these connections

If you find yourself holding back from embracing, as it were, these two connections, it is likely that while you may understand them you don't fully agree with them. In this case, your task is to stand back, identify the doubt, reservation or objection that you have to these connections and then respond to the doubt, etc. Here is an example of how to do this.

Doubt: If I were to hurt my sister's feelings, I would feel guilty no matter what belief I hold about doing so.

Response: When I stand back and look at what I have just said, I can see it as a knee-jerk response. Reviewing the material on the different beliefs underpinning guilt and remorse, I can now see and agree with the idea that while I am bound to feel bad about hurting my sister's feelings, I feel guilty about this because I hold a set of irrational beliefs about doing so. However, if I were to hold a set of rational beliefs about hurting her feelings, I would feel remorse rather than guilt.

Make a commitment to pursue feeling remorse rather than guilt

Make a commitment to pursue feeling remorse rather than guilt and understand that changing your irrational beliefs is the best way of doing this.

I discussed above that you need to see that remorse constitutes the healthy alternative to your guilt feelings at 'C'. After you have done this, you need to make a commitment to work towards this healthy emotion before attempting to question 'A' or change the situation in which the 'A' occurred.

If you want to question 'A' or change the situation, understand that the best time to do this is when you are not disturbed about 'A' or the situation (i.e. when you feel remorse and not guilt) and that your guilt feelings will interfere with your questioning or change attempts. Once you have understood this and that the best way to be undisturbed about 'A' is by thinking rationally about it, you are ready to question your irrational beliefs about 'A'.

The purpose of questioning your beliefs

The purpose of questioning your beliefs is for you to see that your irrational beliefs are irrational and that your rational beliefs are rational. When you question your beliefs (both irrational and rational) your goal is to help yourself see that your irrational beliefs are irrational and your rational beliefs are rational. Strengthening your conviction in your rational belief and weakening your conviction in your irrational belief comes later.

The following table shows the characteristics of both sets of belief, and you should employ these characteristics in your questioning.

Characteristics of irrational beliefs and rational beliefs

Irrational beliefs	Rational beliefs
Rigid or extreme	Flexible or non-extreme
False	True
Illogical	Logical
Leads to unconstructive results	Leads to constructive results

Question both irrational and rational beliefs

As I said above, the purpose of questioning beliefs is to encourage you to see that your irrational beliefs are irrational and that your rational beliefs are rational. This is known as intellectual insight, because while you may understand this point you may not yet have deep conviction in it to the extent that it influences for the better your feelings and behaviour. This 'emotional insight' will come about later and in Chapter 8 I will teach you some techniques to help you in this respect. For you to achieve such intellectual insight, you have to question both your irrational beliefs and your rational beliefs.

Please note that I suggest that, unless there is a good reason not to do so, you always question both your rigid belief and your flexible belief and both your self-depreciation belief and your unconditional self-acceptance belief.

I recommend that you question your rigid belief and your flexible belief together and then question your self-depreciation belief and your unconditional self-acceptance belief also together (see below).

> Question the rigid belief and the alternative flexible belief.
> Question the self-depreciation belief and the alternative unconditional self-acceptance belief.

To illustrate my points, I will continue to use the example of Eric, who said that he would feel guilty about hurting his mother and infuriating his father if he told them that he was going to put his interests before theirs over the coming weekend.

How to question your rigid belief and your flexible belief

Before I show you how to question your rigid and flexible beliefs, let me remind you of their place in guilt and remorse respectively.

Rigid belief → guilt	Flexible belief → remorse
I must not break my moral/ethical code	I don't want to break my moral/ethical code but that does not mean that I must not do so.
I must live up to my moral/ethical code	I would prefer to live up to my moral/ethical code, but I don't have to do so.
I must nor hurt others.	I would prefer not to hurt others, but I am not immune from doing so and I don't have such immunity.

I recommend that you use three main questions when questioning your rigid belief and flexible belief:

- the empirical question
- the logical question
- the pragmatic question.

Then you can ask which belief you want to strengthen and which you want to weaken, and why.

First, focus on your rigid belief and your flexible belief alternative. Write these down side by side (as above). Then move on to the three questions. I will present them in a certain order, but this order is only a guide and other orders are fine.

The empirical question

Ask yourself: Which of the following beliefs is true and which is false, and why?

- my rigid belief
- my flexible belief.

According to REBT theory, the only correct answer to this question is that your flexible belief is true and your rigid belief is false. Note the following:

A rigid belief is inconsistent with reality. For such a belief to be true the rigidly demanded conditions would already have to exist, when they do not. Or as soon as you made your rigid demand then these demanded conditions would have to come into existence. Both positions are patently inconsistent with reality.

On the other hand, a flexible belief is true since its two component parts are true. These two components are an asserted preference and a negated demand. You can prove that you have a particular desire and can provide reasons why you want what you want (asserted preference). You can also prove that you do not have to get what you desire (negated demand).

Eric's example

Question Which of the following beliefs is true and which is false, and why?

> *Rigid belief*: 'I must not hurt my mother and infuriate my father.'
> *Flexible belief*: 'I don't want to hurt my mother and infuriate my father, but sadly it does not follow that I must not do so.'

Answer My flexible belief is true and my rigid belief is false.

My rigid belief that I must not hurt my mother and infuriate my father is inconsistent with reality. The reality is that if I do hurt my mother and infuriate my father then that is what I have done and my demand is my attempt to make reality the way I want it to be. Sadly, I don't have such control! For, if I did, my rigid belief would prevent me from hurting my mother and infuriating my father.

On the other hand, my flexible belief that I don't want to hurt my mother and infuriate my father, but sadly it does not follow that I must not do so, is true. It is certainly true that I don't want to upset them and it is also true that it does not follow that I must not do so.

The logical question

Ask yourself: Which of the following beliefs is logical and which is illogical, and why?

- my rigid belief
- my flexible belief.

According to REBT theory your rigid belief is illogical while your flexible belief is logical. Your rigid belief is based on the same desire as your flexible belief, but you transform it as follows:

> I prefer that *x* happens (or does not happen) . . . and therefore this absolutely must (or must not) happen.

This belief has two components. The first ['I prefer that *x* happens (or does not happen)'] is not rigid, but the second ['. . . and therefore this must (or must not) happen'] is rigid. As such your rigid belief is not logical since one cannot logically derive something rigid from something that is not rigid.

Your flexible belief is as follows:

> I prefer that *x* happens (or does not happen) . . . but this does not mean that it must (or must not) happen.

Your flexible belief is logical since both parts are not rigid and thus the second component logically follows from the first.

Eric's example

Question   Which of the following beliefs is logical and which is illogical, and why?

> *Rigid belief:* 'I must not hurt my mother and infuriate my father.'
> *Flexible belief:* 'I don't want to hurt my mother and infuriate my father, but sadly it does not follow that I must not do so.'

Answer   My flexible belief is logical and my rigid belief is illogical.
My rigid belief, 'I must not hurt my mother and infuriate my father', is illogical. This rigid belief has two components. The first component is based on my preference, 'I don't want to hurt my mother and infuriate my father . . .', and is not rigid. The second component, '. . . and therefore I must not do so', is rigid. Therefore my rigid belief is

illogical since one cannot logically derive something rigid from something that is not rigid.

On the other hand, my flexible belief, 'I don't want to hurt my mother and infuriate my father, but sadly it does not follow that I must not do so', is logical. This flexible belief also has two components. The first component is based on my preference, 'I don't want to hurt my mother and infuriate my father', and is not rigid, The second component, '. . . but sadly it does not follow that I must not do so', is also not rigid. Therefore, my flexible belief is logical since its two components are not rigid and are therefore logically connected together.

The pragmatic question

Ask yourself: Which of the following beliefs leads to largely good results and which leads to largely poor results, and why?

- my rigid belief
- my flexible belief.

You need to acknowledge that your rigid belief leads to unhealthy results for you, while your flexible belief leads to healthier results. Write down the consequences of holding both beliefs and refer, if necessary, to the section entitled 'Understand and agree with the "iB–guilt" and "rB–remorse" connections' on pages 65–6.

Eric's example

Question Which of the following beliefs leads to largely good results and which leads to largely poor results, and why?

Rigid belief: 'I must not hurt my mother and infuriate my father.'
Flexible belief: 'I don't want to hurt my mother and infuriate my father, but sadly it does not follow that I must not do so.'

Answer My flexible belief leads to healthy results, while my rigid belief leads to unhealthy results.

When I believe 'I don't want to hurt my mother and infuriate my father, but sadly it does not follow that I must not do so', I feel remorseful rather than guilty and I am inclined to tell my parents that I am going to put myself first on this occasion.

However, when I believe 'I must not hurt my mother and infuriate my father', I feel guilty and put my parents first.

Make a commitment to belief change

Ask yourself: Which belief do I want to strengthen and which do I want to weaken, and why?

After the questioning you have undertaken, it is very likely that you will decide that you wish to work to strengthen your conviction in your flexible belief and to weaken your conviction in your rigid belief. You 'should' also be able to give coherent reasons for your decision based on your problematic feelings and behaviour and your goals for change.

Eric's example

Question Which belief do I want to strengthen and which do I want to weaken, and why?

Answer I want to strengthen my flexible belief: 'I don't want to hurt my mother and infuriate my father, but sadly it does not follow that I must not do so' because it is true, logical and will help me have a more balanced relationship with my parents, in that we both have an opportunity to get what we want some of the time.

I want to weaken my rigid belief: 'I must not hurt my mother and infuriate my father' because it is false, illogical and will interfere with me developing a more balanced relationship with my parents in the sense that we all have a chance of getting what we want at different times.

How to question your self-depreciation belief and your unconditional self-acceptance belief

Before I show you how to question your self-depreciation belief and unconditional self-acceptance (USA) belief, let me remind you of their place in guilt and remorse respectively.

Self-depreciation belief → guilt	USA belief → remorse
I am a bad person if I break my moral/ethical code	I am not a bad person if I break my moral/ethical code. I'm a fallible human being who has done a wrong thing.
I am rotten if I don't live up to my moral/ethical code.	I am not rotten if I don't live up to my moral/ethical code. I am a unique person who failed to do the right thing.
I am a selfish person if I hurt others.	I am not a selfish person if I hurt others. Rather, I am a complex, fallible human being if I do so.

As I discussed in Chapter 1, guilt involves self-depreciation. Thus, you need to question your self-depreciation and your unconditional self-acceptance beliefs, again using the same three questions that I discussed in the previous section: the empirical question, the logical question and the pragmatic question. As before, once you have done this again ask yourself which belief you want to strengthen and which you want to weaken, and why.

Start off by focusing on your self-depreciation belief and your unconditional self-acceptance belief alternative. Write these down side by side (as above). Then move on to the three questions.

The empirical question

Ask yourself: Which of the following beliefs is true and which is false, and why?

- my self-depreciation belief
- my unconditional self-acceptance belief.

According to REBT theory, an unconditional self-acceptance belief is true and a self-depreciation belief is false.

When you hold a self-depreciation belief you believe *at the time* the following:

- You can legitimately be given a single global rating that defines your essence, and your worth as a person is dependent upon conditions that change (e.g. your worth goes up when you do well and goes down when you don't do well).
- You can be rated on the basis of one of your aspects.

If you stand back, you will see that these convictions are inconsistent with reality and that your unconditional self-acceptance belief is true, since this is made up of the following ideas:

- You cannot legitimately be given a single global rating that defines your essence, and your worth, as far as you have it, is not dependent upon conditions that change (e.g. your worth stays the same whether or not you do well).
- It makes sense to rate discrete aspects of you, but it does not make sense to rate the whole of you on the basis of these discrete aspects.

Eric's example

Question   Which of the following beliefs is true and which is false, and why?

Self-depreciation belief: 'I would be a bad person if I were to hurt my mother and infuriate my father.'
Unconditional self-acceptance belief: 'I would not be a bad person if I were to hurt my mother and infuriate my father. I would be a fallible human being who would be doing something that I do not want to do in order to do something that would be in my healthy interests.'

Answer   My unconditional self-acceptance belief is true and my self-depreciation belief is false.

I can prove that I am the same fallible human being whether I hurt my parents' feelings or not. I am far too complex to be defined by one experience, and my fallibility is fixed and does not depend on whether or not I hurt my parents. So when I say that I would be a bad person if I hurt my mother and infuriated my father I am wrong, since this is inconsistent with reality. If I were bad then I could only do bad things, which is obviously false.

The logical question

Ask yourself: Which of the following beliefs is logical and which is illogical, and why?

• my self-depreciation belief
• my unconditional self-acceptance belief.

According to REBT theory your self-depreciation belief is illogical, while your unconditional self-acceptance belief is logical.

When you hold a self-depreciation belief, this belief is based on the same idea as your self-acceptance belief in that in both you acknowledge that it would be bad if 'A' happened, but you transform it as follows:

'A' is bad . . . and therefore I am bad.

Thus, your self-depreciation belief has two components. The first ('A' is bad . . .) is an evaluation of a part of your experience, while the second (. . . and therefore I am bad) is an evaluation of the whole of your 'self'. As such, you are making the illogical part–whole error where the part is deemed illogically to define the whole.

Your unconditional self-acceptance belief is as follows:

'A' is bad, but this does not mean that I am bad. I am a fallible human being even though 'A' happened.

Your unconditional self-acceptance belief is logical because it shows that your 'self' is complex and incorporates the bad event. Thus, in holding your unconditional self-acceptance belief you avoid making the part–whole error.

Eric's example

Question   Which of the following beliefs is true and which is false, and why?

> *Self-depreciation belief*: 'I would be a bad person if I were to hurt my mother and infuriate my father.'
> *Unconditional self-acceptance belief*: 'I would not be a bad person if I were to hurt my mother and infuriate my father. I would be a fallible human being who would be doing something that I do not want to do in order to do something that would be in my healthy interests.'

Answer   My unconditional self-acceptance belief is logical and my self-depreciation belief is illogical.

It would be bad if I hurt my parents' feelings, but that constitutes an evaluation of one experience. It is therefore part of my life, albeit a small part. To say that I would be bad if this happened is illogical, because in saying this I am stating that one experience can define me as a person. In doing this I am making the part–whole error. On the other hand, when I say that hurting my parents' feelings would not make me worth less and that I would be the same fallible human being whether or not I hurt them, this is logical because in saying this I am recognizing that my 'self' would incorporate this experience and would not be defined by it. I would therefore avoid making the part–whole error.

The pragmatic question

Ask yourself: Which of the following beliefs leads to largely good results and which leads to largely poor results, and why?'

- my self-depreciation belief
- my unconditional self-acceptance belief.

You need to acknowledge that your self-depreciation belief leads to unhealthy results for you, while your unconditional self-acceptance belief leads to healthier results. Write down the consequences of holding both beliefs, and if necessary refer once again to the section entitled 'Understand and agree with the "iB–guilt" and "rB–remorse" connections' that I discussed on pages 65–6.

Question   Which of these beliefs will lead to largely healthy results and which to largely unhealthy results, and why?

Self-depreciation belief: 'I would be a bad person if I were to hurt my mother and infuriate my father.'
Unconditional self-acceptance belief: 'I would not be a bad person if I were to hurt my mother and infuriate my father. Rather, I would be a fallible human being who would be doing something that I do not want to do in order to do something that would be in my healthy interests.'

Answer   My self-depreciation belief will lead largely to unhealthy results, while my unconditional self-acceptance belief will lead to healthy results.

When I believe: 'I would not be a bad person if I were to hurt my mother and infuriate my father. Rather, I would be a fallible human being who would be doing something that I do not want to do in order to do something that would be in my healthy interests', I would feel remorseful rather than guilty and I would be inclined to tell my parents that I am going to put myself first on this occasion.

However, when I believe: 'I would be a bad person if I were to hurt my mother and infuriate my father', I would feel guilty and would put my parents first.

Make a commitment to belief change

Ask yourself: Which belief do I want to strengthen and which do I want to weaken, and why?

After the questioning you have undertaken, you 'should' decide that you wish to work to strengthen your conviction in your unconditional self-acceptance belief and to weaken your conviction in your depreciation belief. You 'should' also be able to give coherent reasons for your decision based on your feelings of hurt and your goals for change.

Eric's example

Question   Which of the following beliefs do I want to strengthen and which do I want to weaken, and why?

Self-depreciation belief: 'I would be a bad person if I were to hurt my mother and infuriate my father.'
Unconditional self-acceptance belief: 'I would not be a bad person if I were to hurt my mother and infuriate my father. Rather, I would be a fallible human being who would be doing something that I do not want to do in order to do something that would be in my healthy interests.'

Answer I want to strengthen my unconditional self-acceptance belief: 'I would not be a bad person if I were to hurt my mother and infuriate my father. Rather, I would be a fallible human being who would be doing something that I do not want to do in order to do something that would be in my healthy interests' because it is true, logical and will help me handle the situation with my parents in a healthier way, both emotionally and behaviourally.

I want to weaken my self-depreciation: 'I would be a bad person if I were to hurt my mother and infuriate my father' because it is false, illogical and will interfere with me handling the situation with my parents in a healthier way, both emotionally and behaviourally.

In the following chapter, I will teach you several techniques designed to help you to strengthen conviction in your remorse-based rational beliefs and to weaken your conviction in your guilt-based irrational beliefs.

8

Deepening conviction in your remorse-based rational beliefs

Introduction

In this chapter, I will teach you a number of techniques devised to help you strengthen your conviction in your rational beliefs and weaken your conviction in your irrational beliefs. Unfortunately, you need to work at truly believing your rational beliefs so that that they make a real difference to the way that you feel and act. Why? Because just understanding that your rational beliefs are consistent with reality and are logical and helpful to you is not sufficient to bring about change. This form of understanding is known as 'intellectual insight', and when you have it you say things such as 'I understand why my rational belief is rational, but I don't believe it yet' or 'I understand that my rational belief is rational up here [referring to your head] but not down here [referring to your gut].' This type of insight is necessary to help you change your rational beliefs, but is not sufficient for you to do so.

The type of insight that promotes change is known by REBT therapists as 'emotional insight'. If you have this type of insight you say things like 'Not only do I believe it in my head, I feel it in my gut' and 'I really believe that my rational belief is true.' The true indicator of whether you have emotional insight into your rational belief is that this belief leads to remorse-based, constructive behaviour (as listed on p. 61) and realistic thinking (as listed on p. 62). In this chapter, I will describe a number of techniques that are designed to help you to believe in your gut what you understand in your head.

The attack–response technique

This technique, which is sometimes called the zigzag technique, is based on the idea that you can strengthen your conviction in a rational belief by responding persuasively to attacks on this belief. There are a number of variations of this technique which I will briefly mention later. But first let me outline the main (written) version of the attack–response technique.

Instructions on how to complete a written attack–response form

Write down your specific remorse-based *rational* belief on a piece of paper.

Rate your present level of conviction in this belief on a scale of 0 to 100, with 0 = no conviction and 100 = total conviction (i.e. 'I really believe this my gut and it markedly influences my feelings and behaviour'). Write down this rating under your belief.

Write down an attack on this rational belief. Your attack may take the form of a doubt, reservation or objection to this rational belief. It should also contain an explicit irrational belief (e.g. rigid belief or self-depreciation belief). Make this attack as genuine as you can. The more it reflects what you believe, the better.

Respond to this attack as fully as you can. It is really important that you respond to each element of the attack. In particular, make sure that you respond to irrational belief statements and also to distorted or unrealistic inferences framed in the form of a doubt, reservation or objection to the rational belief. Do so as persuasively as possible and write down your response.

Continue in this vein until you have answered all of your attacks and cannot think of any more. Make sure throughout this process that you are keeping the focus on the rational belief that you are trying to strengthen.

If you find this exercise difficult, make your attacks gentle at first. Then, when you can respond to these attacks quite easily, begin to make the attacks more biting. Work in this way until you are making really strong attacks. When you make an attack, do so as if you really want to believe it. And when you respond, really throw yourself into it with the intention of demolishing the attack and of strengthening your conviction in your rational belief.

Don't forget that the purpose of this exercise is to strengthen your conviction in your rational belief, so it is important that you stop only when you have answered all of your attacks.

When you have answered all of your attacks, re-rate your level of conviction in your rational belief using the 0–100 scale as before. If you have succeeded in responding persuasively to your attacks, then this rating will have gone up appreciably.

Eric's example

Here is how Eric used the attack–response technique to strengthen his unconditional self-acceptance belief.

Rational belief I would not be a bad person if I were to hurt my mother and infuriate my father. Rather, I would be a fallible human being who would be doing something that I do not want to do in order to do something that will be in my healthy interests. [Conviction rating of rational belief = 20.]

Attack But that's a cop-out. You are trying to excuse your behaviour. You are bad. Saying that you are fallible is ducking the issue.

Response No, it's not a cop-out. I am taking responsibility for my behaviour. I will endeavour to tell my parents as sensitively as possible that, on this occasion, I am going to put myself first. How is saying that I am fallible ducking the issue? It is a fact about me, and you baldly saying that I am bad does not make me bad. Look, the matter is this. I do put my parents first quite a bit of the time and don't do what I want to do. But now, some of the time, I am going to put myself first and that may mean that my mother feels hurt and my father feels infuriated. I am sorry about that, but while it is bad if this happens it does not mean that I am bad. That experience does not and cannot define me.

Attack But you know how your parents are going to react when you tell them that you are going to do what you want to do. After all they have done for you in their lives, what kind of ungrateful, selfish person are you?

Response Yes, I can predict that they are going to be upset. I am well aware that me putting myself first contributes to these feelings. However, it is ludicrous for you to say that I am an ungrateful, selfish person. First, I am grateful for all my parents have done for me over the years. Their example has helped me to do something similar for my son. However, I really dispute the idea that I am a selfish person. I care about my parents and I am sorry that they may well be distressed at me putting myself first on this occasion. I am trying to care for myself as well as care for them and this is hardly being selfish. If I were selfish I would cynically put myself first without caring at all about how my parents feel. This does not describe me at all. I care for my parents and I also care for myself. Does that make me an ungrateful, selfish person? I really don't think so. [Conviction rating of original rational belief = 75.]

Variations of the attack–response technique

I mentioned earlier that there are a number of variations of the attack–response technique. Thus, you can voice-record the dialogue and make sure that your response is more forceful in tone and language than your attack. You can also use the technique with a friend who can make increasingly biting attacks on your rational belief, encouraging you to respond effectively to these attacks. This is often called the devil's advocate technique.

Using rational-emotive imagery

Rational-emotive imagery (REI) is an imagery method designed to help you practise changing your *specific* irrational belief to its healthy equivalent while you imagine, at the same time, focusing on what you are most disturbed about in a *specific* situation in which you felt guilty.

REI is based on the fact that you can use your imagery modality to help you get over your problems with guilt or, albeit unwittingly, to practise thinking unhealthily as you imagine a host of negative situations about which you make yourself feel guilty. In the latter case, when you think about a negative event and you make yourself feel guilty, you are likely to do so by imagining the event in your mind's eye and covertly rehearsing one or more irrational beliefs about the event. In this way, you literally practise making yourself feel guilty and at the same time you end up by strengthening your conviction in your irrational beliefs.

Fortunately, you can also use your mind's eye for constructive purposes. For instance, while imagining the same negative event as above, you can practise changing your feelings of guilt to those of remorse by changing your specific irrational beliefs to specific rational beliefs. What follows is a set of instructions for using REI.

- Take a situation in which you felt guilt and identify the aspect of the situation you felt most guilty about.
  - *Eric's example* Eric chose the situation where he imagined telling his parents that he was going away for the weekend rather than visiting them and that his mother felt hurt and his father felt infuriated about him putting himself first. He was most disturbed about hurting his mother and infuriating his father.
- Close your eyes and imagine the situation as vividly as possible and focus on the adversity at 'A'.
  - *Eric's example* Eric closed his eyes and imagined his parents feeling upset as outlined above. He focused on the idea that he hurt his mother and infuriated his father.
- Allow yourself to really experience the guilt feelings that you felt at the time while still focusing intently on the 'A'.

- *Eric's example*   Eric made himself feel very guilty while focusing on upsetting his parents.
• Really experience your guilt for a moment or two and then change your emotional response to remorse, which is the healthy negative alternative to guilt. While you do this, keep focusing intently on the adversity at 'A'. Do not change the intensity of your guilt; rather, change your feeling to remorse, but keep this feeling as strong as your guilt. Keep experiencing your remorse for about five minutes, all the time focusing on the 'A'. If you go back to your guilt feelings, bring your remorse back.
  - *Eric's example*   Eric kept feeling guilty for a few moments, but then changed his feelings to remorse about hurting his mother and infuriating his father. Initially he had trouble doing this, but eventually did so. He maintained the same level of intensity of his remorse as when he felt guilty.
• At the end of five minutes, ask yourself how you have changed your emotion.
  - *Eric's example*   Eric then asked himself how he managed to change his feelings of guilt about upsetting his parents to feelings of remorse.
• Make sure that you have changed your emotional response from guilt to remorse by changing your specific irrational belief to its healthy alternative. If you did not do so (if, for example, you changed your emotion by changing the 'A' to make it less negative or neutral or by holding an indifference belief about the 'A'), do the exercise again, and keep doing this until you have changed your guilt to remorse only by changing your specific irrational belief to its healthy alternative.
  - *Eric's example*   Eric changed his feelings of guilt about upsetting his parents to feelings of remorse by changing his rigid belief, where he demanded that he must not upset his parents, to his flexible belief, whereby he recognized that it would be unfortunate if he upset his parents, but that he was not immune from doing so and neither did he have to be immune.

My final point about REI concerns how frequently you should practise it. I suggest that you practise it several times a day and aim for 30 minutes of daily practice (when you are not doing any other therapy homework). You might practise it more frequently and for a longer period of time when you are about to face a negative situation about which you are likely to feel guilt. When you are doing other therapy homework, 15 minutes of daily REI practice will suffice.

Teaching your remorse-based rational beliefs to others

Another way of strengthening your conviction in your remorse-based rational beliefs is to teach them to others. I am not suggesting that you play the role of therapist to friends and relatives, nor am I suggesting that you foist these ideas on people who are not interested in discussing them. Rather, I am suggesting that you teach rational beliefs to people who hold the alternative irrational beliefs and are interested in hearing what you have to say on the subject. When you do this, and in particular when the other person argues with your viewpoint in defending his or her position, you get the experience of responding to these arguments with persuasive arguments of your own, and in doing so you strengthen your conviction in your own rational beliefs. I suggest that you do this after you have developed competence at using the written attack–response technique discussed earlier, since the back-and-forth discussion which often ensues when you attempt to teach rational beliefs to others is reminiscent of this technique.

Eric's example

Eric had developed a fair measure of success in developing his rational belief about upsetting his parents when he met up with his sister-in-law, who had just upset her parents and who held a similar irrational belief about upsetting her parents as Eric did. Eric attempted to teach his sister-in-law rational thinking about upsetting her parents. While this did not prove successful, at least in the short term, in that his sister-in-law clung tenaciously to the idea that she absolutely should not have upset her parents, Eric found the experience very valuable in that he could see clearly the holes in the arguments which his sister-in-law used to defend her own irrational belief. In coming up with rational counter-arguments to his sister-in-law's points, Eric developed greater conviction in his own rational beliefs about upsetting his parents.

Use of rational self-statements

Once you have developed your specific rational beliefs, you can develop shorthand versions of these beliefs which you can write down on a small card or, as one of my clients does, type them into the message folder of your mobile phone and review them periodically. Such review is especially useful, both when you are about to face an adversity and while you are actually facing one, assuming that it is feasible to glance at your rational message. You can also repeat these self-statements to yourself in a forceful, persuasive manner. When you repeat such rational self-statements, do so mindfully. A mindless repetition will have no impact on your feelings or behaviour.

Eric's example

Eric constructed the following rational self-statements which helped him to increase conviction in his developing rational beliefs about upsetting his parents:

- 'I'm not immune from upsetting my parents, even though I'd really like to be.'
- 'I am not bad when I upset my parents. I'm fallible.'
- 'I don't always have to put my parents first.'

Rehearse your rational beliefs while acting and thinking in ways that are consistent with these beliefs

Perhaps the most powerful way of strengthening your remorse-based rational belief is to rehearse it while facing the relevant adversity at 'A' and while acting and thinking in ways that are consistent with this rational belief. When all these systems are working together in sync and you keep them in sync repeatedly, you maximize your chances of strengthening your conviction in your rational belief. Conversely, refrain from acting and thinking in ways that are consistent with your old irrational belief. This will be difficult for you because you are used to acting and thinking in unconstructive ways when your irrational belief is activated. However, if you monitor your belief, your behaviour and your subsequent thinking, and respond constructively to all three when you identify them, then you will go against your tendency (1) to evaluate yourself, others and/or the world in rigid and extreme terms (belief), (2) to act self-defeatingly (behaviour) and (3) to think unrealistically (subsequent thinking). If you do this successfully, then you will gain valuable experience at weakening your conviction in your irrational beliefs and strengthening your conviction in your rational beliefs.

You need to set yourself homework tasks designed to help you to do the above. In doing so it is important for you to acknowledge the following.

You may have been employing a number of safety-seeking strategies designed to help you avoid facing adversities or to protect yourself psychologically if you have to face these adversities. Continued use of these strategies while you are endeavouring to change your irrational beliefs will undermine your attempts to do so. So, identify these safety-seeking strategies (which are largely behavioural and thinking in nature and can often be subtle and difficult to spot) and question the irrational beliefs that often underpin them, so that you can face the adversities fairly and squarely while rehearsing your developing rational beliefs and while acting and thinking in ways that are not safety-seeking in purpose.

You will not experience a change in your unhealthy guilt feelings until after much integrated practice at holding to your rational beliefs and acting and thinking in ways that are consistent with these beliefs. Thus, emotional change tends to lag behind behavioural change and thinking change. If you understand this, then you will persist at changing your thinking and behaviour and will not get discouraged when your guilt feelings take longer to change.

It is important that you face negative events about which you feel guilt so that you can practise your rational beliefs and the constructive thinking and acting that stem from these beliefs. As you do so, face events that pose a challenge to your developing rational beliefs and related thoughts and behaviour, but which you do not find overwhelming for you.

Eric's example

To help himself act and think in ways consistent with his rational belief and refrain from acting and thinking in ways consistent with his irrational belief, Eric first listed these behaviours and thoughts under their respective headings as follows:

Rational belief

'I don't want to hurt my mother and infuriate my father, but sadly it does not follow that I must not do so. I would not be a bad person if I were to do so. I would be a fallible human being who would be doing something that I do not want to do in order to do something that would be in my healthy interests.'

Actions consistent with my rational belief
- Telling my parents that I am going to put myself first at times and put them first at other times and that I am remorseful if they are upset about this.
- Asking my mother why she gets hurt when I tell her that I want to put myself first and discussing the matter with her.
- Asking my father why he gets infuriated when I tell him that I want to put myself first and discussing the matter with him.

Subsequent thoughts consistent with my rational belief
- Thinking of ways to express my remorse to my parents about upsetting them.

Irrational belief

'I must not hurt my mother and infuriate my father. I would be a bad person if I were to hurt my mother and infuriate my father.'

Actions consistent with my irrational belief
- Putting my parents first.
- Not discussing my feelings with my parents.

Subsequent thoughts consistent with my irrational belief
- Thinking of ways of avoiding my parents.
- Thinking obsessively of a solution where I do what I want without upsetting my parents.

After making these two lists, Eric resolved to rehearse his rational belief and think and act in the ways he had identified as being consistent with this belief, and did so whenever he could. He first imagined speaking to his parents before actually doing it, and as he did so he rehearsed his rational belief.

Eric also refrained from acting and thinking in ways he had identified as being consistent with his irrational belief. When he felt like acting and thinking in these ways, he used these urges to go back and question his irrational belief and remind himself why this belief is false, illogical and unproductive. He then reviewed his rational belief and the reasons why it is true, sensible and helpful to him.

In these ways, Eric strengthened his conviction in his rational belief and weakened his conviction in his irrational belief.

After he had prepared for the encounter as discussed above, Eric spoke to his parents about his wish to put himself first and his remorse about hurting their feelings. As predicted, his parents were upset with Eric and his father, in particular, called him selfish for the stance he was taking. Eric told his father that he felt sorry his father thought he was selfish and argued his point that he was trying to ensure they all had an opportunity of getting something of what they wanted, rather than the previous position where he put his parents first all the time.

Understanding how your mind works when you feel guilty and are trying to change

I showed you in Chapter 2 that when you hold guilt-related irrational beliefs at 'B' then these beliefs influence your subsequent thinking at 'C' in the 'ABC' framework. Such thinking is characterized by being highly distorted and skewed to the negative (see pp. 13–16). I discussed in Chapter 3 that when you hold an alternative set of remorse-related rational beliefs at 'B', these beliefs also influence your subsequent thinking at 'C', but in a different way. Such thinking is characterized by being balanced and realistic.

Now, when you are working to strengthen conviction in your rational beliefs and weaken conviction in your irrational beliefs, your subsequent thinking at 'C' may be slow to change. This means that you may still have highly distorted guilt-related thoughts at 'C' when you are practising your rational beliefs at 'B'. It is important to remember that when you are doing so, your conviction in your irrational beliefs is still likely to be strong and these irrational beliefs will lead to highly distorted thinking.

When such highly distorted thoughts come into your mind while you are rehearsing your rational beliefs, it is important that you understand that this is how your mind works when you try to change. I suggest that you do the following: acknowledge the existence of such thoughts without trying to suppress them, distract yourself from them or engage with them. This is known as the acceptance strategy. If you find it difficult to grasp the idea of having a thought without engaging with it, here is an analogy that you may find helpful.

Imagine that you are walking down a high street and a charity worker approaches you and tries to engage you in a conversation about a local charity. You know that he (in this case) wants you to sign a direct debit form whereby you pay a regular sum every month to the charity. Now, let's suppose that you want neither to give to the charity nor to talk to the person. What is the best way of stopping the person from talking to you without being overtly rude to him? My view is that the best way to do this is not to respond to the person. As you continue down the road, the charity worker walks beside you and you are aware of what he is saying but you say nothing in return. You give the person no eye contact and show him no recognition that he is there. If you take this tack, after a short while the person will stop pursuing you. This is the approach you need to take with your safety-seeking thoughts. Acknowledge that they are present, but continue with what you are doing while not engaging with the thoughts and without trying to get rid of them.

If relevant, use the presence of such thinking to identify and deal with the irrational beliefs that are still active.

Question the empirical nature of these thinking 'C's once or twice (see Chapter 10, p. 108 for suggestions about how to do this) and then return to the acceptance strategy detailed above.

Eric's example

While striving to rehearse his remorse-based rational beliefs about hurting his parents, Eric was aware that thoughts about being punished for hurting his parents still came into his mind. He understood why he still had such thoughts and did not engage with them. He saw having such thoughts as akin to having an after-image of a light bulb after staring at it for a long time. As he continued to rehearse his rational beliefs and acted in ways consistent with them, such distorted thoughts faded from his mind.

Epilogue

After using the methods described in this part of the book, Eric now feels remorseful, but not guilty, about this and similar episodes where his parents felt upset about Eric putting himself first. As a consequence, he is not consumed with guilt when he does put himself first and at times still puts his parents first. Eventually, his parents came to accept this state of affairs although they never came to like it.

9

Dealing with lapses in guilt and preventing relapse

Introduction

Having made progress in developing your remorse response, it is vital to deal with lapses to continued progress and to prevent any relapse. I regard a lapse, in this context, as a temporary non-serious return to a state where you go back to experiencing guilt. A relapse, on the other hand, is a more permanent and serious return to that state. To prevent such a relapse I suggest you follow the relapse prevention sequence.

The relapse prevention sequence and how to use it

Remember that the following sequence of steps for ensuring prevention of relapse and the order in which I have presented them are a suggestion and you do not need to follow them slavishly. They should be used as a guide, which you can modify to suit your own circumstances.

Step 1: Review your present achievement in developing remorse

This first step in the relapse prevention sequence relates to your progress up until now in developing your remorse response. To take effective action in dealing with your relapse you first need to appreciate what you have achieved so far. You may also find it helpful to think back on what you have learned that has enabled you to progress in your development of remorse as a healthy alternative to guilt.

Step 2: Think through how you can apply what you have learnt to future situations to which you could respond with remorse

Using the knowledge acquired from Step 1 you can now begin to think through how you may be able to apply this learning to problems you may encounter in the future where you may break your moral/ethical code, fail to live up to your moral/ethical code or hurt others' feelings.

Step 3: Develop rational beliefs about lapses

At the beginning of this chapter I defined a lapse as a temporary and non-serious return to a state where you go back to feeling guilt. It is quite likely that you will experience a number of such lapses in your journey to developing remorse. What is important is that you develop rational beliefs about experiencing such lapses. By doing so you will learn from them.

On the other hand, if you have a set of irrational beliefs about lapsing then you may disturb yourself about doing so, and this will prevent you from learning from these lapses, thus increasing the chances of experiencing a relapse (which I define as a more enduring, serious return to a state where you routinely respond to acts of moral commission and omission and hurting others with guilt).

The following is a set of rational beliefs which you can adapt for your own use in thinking about and responding to the lapses that will inevitably occur on your journey to developing your remorse response.

- I would rather not experience lapses in responding with remorse, but I am not immune from them, nor do I have to be.
- It is unfortunate to experience lapses in responding with remorse, but it isn't the end of the world.
- It is a struggle to tolerate lapses in responding with remorse, but I can put up with them and it is worth it to me to do so.
- I am a fallible human being. I will experience lapses along the way to developing remorse and doing so doesn't make me less of a person.
- Lapses in responding with remorse don't make the world a rotten place. The world is a complex mixture of the good, the bad and the neutral.

If you develop this kind of rational philosophy, you will be in the best position to deal with the main reason people relapse – failure to deal with the factors that make them especially liable to lapse in the first place.

Step 4: Identify factors to which you remain vulnerable

Vulnerability factors are factors that, if you encounter them, lead you to be vulnerable to respond with guilt to moral commissions, omissions and situations where you have hurt people. Such a vulnerability factor may be external or internal to you. A typical external vulnerability factor would be others directly accusing you of hurting their feelings. So, if you want to do something and others who are involved accuse you of not caring for them and being selfish, this may well represent an external vulnerability factor for you.

Internal vulnerability factors are factors inside you which you regard as evidence of immorality, for example. In particular, people who are prone to guilt find experiencing certain thoughts and urges which they regard as forbidden particularly guilt-provoking (e.g. finding an under-age girl sexually attractive).

The most reliable method for identifying a vulnerability factor is to think back over times when you lapsed back into guilt, having made progress. If such lapses occurred in situations that resembled each other, then a vulnerability factor is likely to be present.

Malcolm's example

Malcolm, for instance, had been doing very well in dealing with his guilt about leaving work on time without feeling guilty, something that he had found particularly difficult previously. However, he noticed that he had recently begun to stay at work longer and longer. On assessing his problem, he noticed that he started to do this when a new colleague began to stay late at work. Malcolm concluded that his vulnerable factor was as follows: 'It would be very selfish of me to leave work on time when my new colleague is working late.'

Step 5: Use the 'situational ABC' model in dealing with vulnerability factors

In Chapter 5, I outlined CBT's 'situational ABC' model that you can use to assess and deal with your guilt. You can also use this model to deal with your vulnerability factors as follows:

- Describe the situation in which your vulnerability factor occurred.
- Specify your responses at 'C' which would include (1) an unhealthy negative emotion – guilt; (2) an unconstructive behaviour or action tendency; and, if relevant, (3) a highly distorted thought or thoughts, with a negative bias.
- Remind yourself of your vulnerability factor at 'A'.
- Identify the irrational beliefs at 'B' that underlie the above responses at 'C'. State your rigid belief and your self-depreciation belief.
- State the responses at 'C' that demonstrate what you are aiming for when meeting your vulnerability factor at 'A'. Assuming that the vulnerability factor is a negative event, your emotional goal will be negative but healthy (i.e. remorse), your behavioural goal will be constructive and your thinking goal will be realistic.
- Identify those rational beliefs at 'B' that underlie your emotional, behavioural and thinking goals. Specify your flexible belief and your unconditional self-acceptance belief.
- Examine your rational and irrational beliefs by questioning them

until it is clear to you that the former are true, logical and helpful and the latter are false, illogical and unhelpful.
• Make a commitment to yourself to strengthening your rational beliefs.

This is how Malcolm used the 'situational ABC' model' to help him deal with his vulnerability factor. In the first 'situational ABC', I outline his guilt response and in the second I outline his remorse response.

Malcolm's guilt response to his vulnerability factor

Situation 'It is time to leave work when I notice my new colleague is working late.'
'A' (vulnerability factor) 'It would be very selfish of me to leave work on time when my new colleague is working late.'
'B' 'I must not act selfishly and if I do I am a selfish person.'
'C' (emotional) Guilt.
(behavioural) Staying late at work.
(thinking) 'It would be really wrong to leave work when my new colleague is working late.'

Malcolm's remorse response to his vulnerability factor

Situation 'It is time to leave work when I notice my new colleague is working late.'
'A' (vulnerability factor) 'It would be very selfish of me to leave work on time when my new colleague is working late.'
'B' 'I would prefer not to act selfishly, but that does not mean that I must not do so. I am not a selfish person if I leave on time. I am a fallible human being who may be acting selfishly.'
'C' (emotional) Remorse.
(behavioural) Leaving work on time.
(thinking) 'While from one perspective it may be selfish to leave work on time when my new colleague is staying late, from another perspective I am looking after myself by doing so, and I am not responsible for my colleague's choice.'

Malcolm then questioned his beliefs and committed himself to strengthening his rational belief.

Step 6: Use imagery rehearsal of rational beliefs

Having committed yourself to reinforcing the rational beliefs that underlie your desired remorse response to your vulnerability factor, the next step is to make your rational beliefs stronger, especially by the use of rational-emotive imagery (REI), in the following way.

- Close your eyes, imagine yourself facing your vulnerability factor and feel yourself becoming guilty while you do so. Assume temporarily that your 'A' is true.
- While you still face the vulnerability factor, change your emotional response to remorse and maintain that response for a few minutes.
- Make sure that you have changed your emotional response by exchanging your irrational beliefs for their rational belief equivalents. If you have not, repeat the technique until you have done so.

Repeat this exercise three times a day until your responses to the vulnerability factor indicate remorse rather than guilt.

Malcolm's example

This is how Malcolm used REI to strengthen his rational beliefs.

He closed his eyes and saw himself leaving work on time when his new colleague had decided to work late and focused on his selfish behaviour. In doing so he made himself feel guilt about his behaviour which he assumed temporarily was selfish.

While still focusing on his selfish behaviour, he changed guilt to remorse and maintained that response for a few minutes.

Malcolm then made sure that he changed his emotional response by changing his irrational belief (i.e. 'I must not act selfishly and if I do I am a selfish person') to his rational belief equivalent (i.e. 'I would prefer not to act selfishly, but that does not mean that I must not do so. I am not a selfish person if I leave on time. I am a fallible human being who may be acting selfishly').

Malcolm repeated this exercise three times a day until his responses to the vulnerability factor became more characterized by remorse rather than guilt.

Step 7: Use imagery rehearsal of constructive behaviour

You can also use imagery to rehearse seeing yourself act in ways that are consistent with your remorse-based rational beliefs when facing your vulnerability factor. Some people find this a very useful step before taking action in relation to their actual vulnerability factor, while for others this step is not necessary and might even be counter-productive. You may wish to try out this technique to determine for yourself whether or not it is likely to be helpful to you as a preparation for taking remorse-based action in the real world.

If you decide to use imagery rehearsal to imagine yourself acting in a way consistent with your remorse-based rational beliefs in facing your vulnerability factor, then the more vividly you can imagine doing so, the better. You should bear in mind, however, that some people do not experience vivid imagery, and if this applies to you don't worry, since you can still use this imagery technique to your benefit in the following way:

- Select a vulnerability factor that is challenging for you to deal with, but which you don't find overwhelming.
- Be clear in your mind what your vulnerability factor is. It will probably be the 'A' in the 'situational ABC' framework.
- Be clear in your mind how you are going to deal constructively with this vulnerability factor.
- Choose a situation in which it is likely that you will encounter your vulnerability factor.
- Get yourself into the right frame of mind by rehearsing your relevant rational beliefs.
- Imagine yourself facing your vulnerability factor and dealing with it constructively. It is better to see yourself struggling than to see yourself showing unrealistic mastery.

Repeat this imagery exercise three times a day until you are ready to face the vulnerability in real life.

Malcolm's example

This is how Malcolm used this technique.

He imagined a scenario in which his boss asked him to work late with his new colleague on an evening where he had agreed to meet his friends for an early evening meal. In doing this he focused on the guilt he would feel if he said no. This situation was challenging for him to deal with, but not overwhelming, and it represented his vulnerability factor, the 'A' (i.e. selfishness).

Malcolm was clear in his mind that he was not going to agree to stay late at work. He got himself into the right frame of mind by rehearsing his relevant rational beliefs, i.e. 'I am fallible for acting selfishly. I am not selfish.'

He pictured himself turning down his boss, even though he felt very uncomfortable about doing so when he imagined that everyone, including himself, would think he was acting selfishly. He saw himself wavering as his boss put him under pressure, but in the end he saw himself declining and leaving work on time.

He repeated this imagery exercise three times a day until he was ready to face the vulnerability factor in reality.

Step 8: Put this constructive plan into action by facing your vulnerability factors

Now you have your rational beliefs and a clear idea of how you're going to act, you are ready to face your vulnerability factor. You can use the principle that I have called 'challenging, but not overwhelming', according to which you decide that facing your vulnerability factor in a given context constitutes a challenge for you, but is not overwhelming, You are not, so to speak, biting off more than you can chew by taking this step.

It is useful to get yourself in the right frame of mind by rehearsing your rational belief before you take action and to hold this belief in mind while taking action. Although the former is nearly always possible, the latter is more difficult, given that you may have to concentrate fully on what you are doing and may not have time to rehearse your rational belief, even briefly, when faced with the reality of the situation. Don't worry if this is the case, since your pre-action rehearsal of your rational belief will often be enough to sustain you; if it isn't, you can review and learn from this experience later.

Malcolm's example

This is how Malcolm used this principle in action. He was at work when his boss came over to him and asked him to stay late that night with his colleague to do an urgent piece of work that had to be ready the next day. Before, he would have agreed, but as he was starting to work on his vulnerability factors he replied that he would give it some thought. Malcolm went to the toilet to rehearse his rational beliefs and them came back and told his boss that while he wanted to be helpful, he had plans for the evening and was not prepared to cancel them. He said that he realized he might be acting selfishly, but that was his decision.

Malcolm then left work on time and noticed that both his boss and his colleague did not say goodbye. He told himself that he did not need their approval and that while it was difficult to put himself first in the circumstances, he was not a selfish person. He then reminded himself that while he might be acting selfishly from one perspective, from another perspective he was looking after himself, and that it was important his boss stopped relying on him to stay late.

Step 9: Review your experiences of dealing with these vulnerability factors and learn from these reviews

Once you have taken action in the face of your vulnerability factors several times, you should stand back and review your experiences of doing so in order to learn from them. You will thus be able to fine-tune your responses to your vulnerability factors.

Malcolm's example

Malcolm did this and realized that what was particularly helpful to him in leaving work on time was saying to his boss and his colleague that, while it was difficult for him to say no to working late, it was important to him to learn to look after himself, and that he hoped they would understand, but they did not have to do so. Stating this rational belief out loud to them served as a reminder of it to himself. It also served to remind him that practising self-care was something that he really wanted to do.

Step 10: Develop rational beliefs about relapse

As mentioned at the start of this chapter, a relapse is a more enduring, serious return to guilt – to put it in plain terms, going back to square one. The steps discussed so far have been those you need to take to deal with lapses and your vulnerability factors, which will thus help prevent a relapse. However, as you may relapse when it comes to exercising your remorse-based rational beliefs, it is important for you to address this possibility. Having done so, ask yourself what particular aspect of relapsing in terms of your guilt you would disturb yourself about. This represents your 'A' in the 'situational ABC' framework. In my experience, people disturb themselves about two major 'A's:

1 *Weakness* 'If I relapse in terms of guilt, it will reveal that I have a weakness.'
2 *Loss of self-control* 'If I relapse in terms of my guilt, it shows that I have lost self-control.'

Develop rational beliefs about weakness-related relapse

When you disturb yourself about relapsing because you assume it reveals a weakness in you, you may experience shame, which will motivate you to avoid dealing with the possibility of relapse. You may also think that people will look down on you and dismiss you should you relapse.

If you experience shame about relapsing it's important for you to adopt the following rational beliefs which you should express in your own words.

> *Flexible belief:* 'I really don't want to be weak and relapse, but sadly and regretfully I am not immune from doing so; nor is there any need for me to be so immune.'

Non-awfulizing belief: 'If I were to be weak and relapse, while it would be unfortunate it would not be the end of the world.'

Discomfort tolerance belief: 'I may find it difficult to put up with being weak and relapsing, but I am prepared to tolerate it and it will be worth it to me to do so.'

Unconditional self-acceptance belief: 'It would be bad if I were to relapse, but it wouldn't prove that I'm a weak or pathetic person. It simply means that I am a complex, fallible human being.'

Develop rational beliefs about relapse related to loss of self-control

If you disturb yourself about relapsing because it suggests that you have experienced a loss of self-control, you may tend to experience anxiety which could lead you to make a desperate attempt to regain such self-control. However, given that your attempt is based on desperation it may lead you to become more anxious rather than less anxious, thus increasing the negativity of your subsequent thoughts about the extent and implications of such a loss of self-control (i.e. your subsequent thinking will become highly distorted and skewed to the negative).

If you experience anxiety about the loss of self-control that accompanies relapse, then it's important that you develop the following rational beliefs which, again, you should express in your own words.

Flexible belief: 'I really don't want to relapse and lose self-control, but sadly and regretfully I am not immune from doing so, nor is there any need for me to be immune.'

Non-awfulizing belief: 'If I were to relapse and lose-self-control, while it would be unfortunate it would not be the end of the world.'

Discomfort tolerance belief: 'I may find it difficult to put up with relapsing and losing self-control, but I am prepared to tolerate it and it will be worth it to me to do so.'

Life-acceptance belief: 'It would be bad if I were to relapse and lose self-control, but it wouldn't prove that life is all bad for allowing this to happen to me. Life is a complex mixture of the good, the bad and the neutral.'

Develop rational beliefs about relapse in general

In the two sections above, I have dealt with two of the most common problems that people tend to have about relapsing with respect to guilt (i.e. being weak and losing self-control) and I have outlined the rational beliefs you need to develop if you experience one or both of these issues. However, some people disturb themselves about the act of relapsing itself, and if this applies to you it will be important for you to develop a set of rational beliefs about the fact of relapse itself in the area of inner strength. I will list these here, but suggest that you modify them to suit your own situation.

> *Flexible belief*: 'I really don't want to relapse, but sadly and regretfully I am not immune from it, nor is there any need for me to be immune.'
> *Non-awfulizing belief*: 'If I were to relapse, while it would be unfortunate, it would not be the end of the world.'
> *Discomfort tolerance belief*: 'I may find it difficult to put up with relapsing, but I am prepared to tolerate it and it will be worth it to me to do so.'
> *Unconditional self-acceptance belief*: 'It would be bad if I were to relapse, but it wouldn't prove that I am a weak, pathetic person. It means that I am a complex, fallible human being.'
> *Life-acceptance belief*: 'Life isn't bad if I relapse. It is a complex place where many good, bad and neutral things happen, including relapse.'

Step 11: Learn from relapse

If you develop and implement a rational philosophy about relapsing back into guilt, then you will calm down about the prospect of it happening. This will help you put the likelihood of your relapsing into perspective and also help you realize that you will lessen the chance of doing so if you are diligent in learning from your relapses and deal sufficiently with your vulnerability factors.

Your rational philosophy will also help you learn from the experience of a relapse into guilt should this, in fact, happen to you. It will help you to review times where your guilt-related lapses became more serious and what you should preferably have done to deal with these effectively, thus reducing the chances that you would relapse. Then you would implement this learning, thus helping you to protect yourself from relapsing in future.

Summary

In any process of personal change, it is important to accept that lapses are an inevitable part of this process. I consider developing rational beliefs about lapses as the best way to deal with them. Moreover, to prevent relapse it is important to deal with and learn from your lapses. Most importantly, relapse prevention depends on your identifying and dealing effectively with your vulnerability factors. You can prepare yourself to face your vulnerability factors by using the 'situational ABC' framework and by employing imagery. When you face your vulnerability factors in real life, you can use the 'challenging, but not overwhelming' concept and rehearse relevant rational beliefs before and during the experience. As is the case with lapses, it is best to develop rational beliefs about relapse. If you do, you are less likely to relapse than if you hold irrational beliefs about it. However, if you do relapse, rather than disturb yourself about this grim reality, learn from it.

In the next and final chapter, I will show you how you can become less prone to guilt if you are particularly susceptible to this destructive emotion.

10

How to become less prone to guilt

Introduction

This chapter is written for those who are particularly prone to guilt and who wish to become less prone to this destructive emotion. If you are unsure whether or not this applies to you consult pp. 20–3. If it does apply, I suggest that you put into practice some or all of the following points that are designed to help you become less prone to guilt.

Acknowledge that you are prone to guilt and that it is a problem for you

Once you have understood the nature of guilt (see Chapter 2 for a review) it is important that you do two things before you proceed. First, decide whether you are prone to guilt; re-reading pp. 20–3 will be particularly helpful here. If you are, the second step is for you to decide whether being thus prone is a problem for you that you would like to change. I covered this issue in Chapter 4 and I refer you to this chapter concerning how to do it.

Take responsibility for being prone to guilt

You may acknowledge that you are prone to guilt and see clearly that it is a problem for you which you would like to change, but unless you take responsibility for being prone to guilt you will not be effective in becoming less prone to it. Taking responsibility for your guilt means fully acknowledging that while breaking your moral/ethical code, failing to live up to your moral/ethical code or hurting others will contribute to you feeling guilt, these facts/inferences at 'A' do not and cannot, on their own, cause you to feel guilty. Rather, it is the irrational beliefs that you hold about these 'A's that largely explain why you feel guilt. Taking responsibility for being prone to guilt means fully acknowledging that you hold such irrational beliefs in a variety of different situations and/or about a number of different people.

Taking such responsibility is an important step in becoming less prone to guilt. Without taking this step you will continue to be prone to guilt because you will have done nothing to change the irrational beliefs that underpin your proneness.

Acknowledge that remorse is the healthy alternative to guilt

Once you have taken responsibility for your proneness to guilt and wish to become less prone, the next step is for you to set an appropriate goal for change. It is no good working to overcome your feelings of guilt unless you have a clear idea of what you are going to experience instead and this alternative emotion is acceptable to you. If either of these two conditions is absent then you will make it much harder for yourself to become less prone to guilt. Thus, if you cannot see any alternative to guilt you will tend to think that you are bound to experience it. If you see that remorse is *an* alternative to guilt but is not an acceptable one, then you will not work towards experiencing it.

Before you take this step, review Chapter 3, which is devoted to outlining the nature of remorse. Then, when you are clear that you have understood why remorse is healthy for you, you are ready to take the next step.

Commit yourself to remorse

After you have fully understood that remorse is the constructive alternative to guilt, it is important that you make a commitment to work towards experiencing this emotion when you face a situation where you have, or think you have, broken your moral/ethical code, failed to live up to such a code or hurt others. You might find it helpful to make a written commitment to this effect and to review this every day. Also, you might consider telling a close friend that you are going to work towards experiencing remorse rather than guilt, if you consider that this verbal commitment will help you to do the work necessary to achieve your goal.

Dealing with emotional problems about guilt

One of the reasons you may not work on your guilt problem is that you may have an emotional problem about your guilt. If you have, then this will have the effect of taking you away from dealing with your guilt problem since you will be preoccupied with your disturbed feelings about your guilt. This is known in CBT as meta-disturbance (literally disturbance about disturbance). It is important to assess carefully the nature of this meta-disturbance about guilt so that you can best deal with it.

Assess and deal with emotional problems about guilt

The best way to start dealing with the assessment of any emotional problem you might have about guilt is to ask yourself the question: 'How do I feel about my feeling of guilt?' The most common emotional problems that people have about guilt are as follows: anxiety, depression, shame and unhealthy self-anger. I suggest that you consult my book *Transforming Eight Deadly Emotions into Healthy Ones* (Sheldon Press, 2012) for assistance in how best to deal with such meta-disturbance.

Accept yourself for being prone to guilt

One of the major emotional problems that will interfere with you capitalizing on your commitment to become less prone to guilt at this point is based on your attitude of self-depreciation for being prone to guilt. When you depreciate yourself, you rate your entire 'self' on the basis of this proneness, and this will lead you to feel an unhealthy negative emotion such as shame. Depreciating yourself for being prone to guilt has two main effects. It does nothing to make you any less prone to this destructive emotion and gives you two emotional problems for the price of one: your original guilt, and shame for experiencing such guilt.

If this applies to you it is important that you work towards accepting yourself unconditionally for being prone to guilt. You do this by seeing that your proneness does not define your 'self', but is a part of your fallibility and complexity as a human being. Accepting yourself for being prone to guilt will enable you to focus on the factors that make you thus prone and will encourage you to do something constructive about it (such as following the guidelines in this book) rather than resigning yourself to it. Unconditional self-acceptance, therefore, promotes constructive action and discourages passivity and resignation.

Keep working on specific episodes of guilt

In Chapters 6–8, I outlined the steps that you need to take when working on specific episodes of guilt. In particular, I showed you how to identify what you are most guilty about and how to assess, question and change the irrational beliefs that underpin your situationally based guilt. I recommend that you do this as soon as you notice that you are making yourself feel guilty. Initially, you will need to do this on paper, but after much practice you will be able to do it in your head. You will also be more able to anticipate situations in which you are likely to make yourself feel guilty and to deal productively with your guilt-related irrational beliefs before they take hold and lead to feelings of guilt.

Identify and make use of recurring patterns in your specific examples of guilt

Once you have worked through a number of specific examples of your guilt, you will be able to identify recurring patterns in these specific examples. Thus, you may find that your guilt is mainly about you breaking your moral or ethical codes. If so, make a note of the codes that you consider you have broken when you feel guilty. Or you may find that your guilt is largely about hurting others, in which case make a note of the people whose feelings you think you have hurt when you feel guilty.

Once you have identified recurring patterns in the specific episodes that you have worked on, you can use this information in two main ways. First, you can utilize this information when you work to prevent the occurrence of guilt in vulnerable situations, and second, this information will come in handy when you come to identify the general irrational beliefs that help to explain why you are prone to guilt.

Identify, challenge and change your general guilt-related irrational beliefs

General guilt-related irrational beliefs are irrational beliefs that are general in nature and account for your feelings of guilt across situations. Let me give you some common examples of such beliefs:

- I must always act morally/ethically and if I don't that proves that I am bad.
- I must always put others first and if I don't I am a selfish person.
- I must ensure in my dealings with people that I don't hurt their feelings. If I don't, I am a rotten person.

You challenge your general irrational beliefs in the same way as you learned to challenge your specific irrational beliefs. Thus, you take one of your general irrational beliefs and ask yourself and answer the following questions:

- Is this belief true or false?
- Is this belief logical/sensible or illogical/nonsensical?
- Is this belief helpful or unhelpful?

At this point, you might find it beneficial to review the material on questioning specific irrational beliefs which can be found in Chapter 7. Continue this line of questioning until you clearly understand that your general irrational beliefs are false, illogical and unconstructive.

Next, develop rational alternatives to these general irrational beliefs as follows:

- I want to always act morally/ethically, but sadly I don't have to do so. If I don't, it does not prove I am bad. It proves that I am an ordinary human being who has done the wrong thing.
- I would like to always put others first, but it is not necessary for me to do so. If I don't, I am not a selfish person. I am a fallible human being who has acted selfishly on this occasion.
- It is preferable if I ensure that in my dealings with people I don't hurt their feelings, but I don't have to be successful in this regard. If I'm not, I am not a rotten person. Rather, I am a non-rotten person who has done a rotten thing.

Once you have developed general rational beliefs, question them in the same way as you questioned your general irrational beliefs. Do this until you clearly understand that your general rational beliefs are true, logical and constructive.

Having done this, I suggest that you use the attack–response technique to deepen your conviction in your general rational beliefs (see pp. 79–81 for instructions concerning how to implement this technique).

Accept yourself unconditionally for falling from 'grace'

If you are particularly prone to guilt, it is important that you strive towards unconditional self-acceptance for falling from 'grace'. I define 'grace' as a state where you always do the right thing and never hurt anybody's feelings in your dealings with them. Of course, as a human being with flaws and failings, it is very unlikely that you will never fall from 'grace' and it is important that you accept this grim fact of life, not demand that you must never fall from 'grace', and accept yourself unconditionally when you do so.

In order to accept yourself unconditionally when you fall from 'grace' and thus become less prone to guilt, it is important that you show yourself that your morality and not hurting others are not actually related to your goodness or badness as a person, unless you choose to make them a moral worth issue.

Put somewhat differently, acting morally and not hurting others may well be good things to do, but such behaviours do not make you a good person and, conversely, acting immorally and hurting others may well be bad, but such behaviours do not make you a bad person. Your moral worth as a person, to the extent that you have it, is constant, whereas your behaviour is variable.

As a human being you have great complexity and your worth as a person should reflect this. When you think you are a better person if you act morally, for example, or a worse person if you act immorally, then you are not doing justice to your complexity.

When you rate yourself on the basis of an aspect of yourself, you are making the part–whole error. This is where you use your rating of an aspect of yourself (e.g. your moral behaviour) as a rating of your whole self (i.e. you are a better person if you act morally and a worse person if you act immorally). When you accept yourself unconditionally as an unrateable, complex, unique, fallible human being who is constantly in flux, you do not make the part–whole error because you acknowledge that whether or not you act morally, you are the same person who either has acted morally or has acted immorally.

Once you base your moral worth on the morality or immorality of your behaviour, then you will 'feel' temporarily good about yourself when you act morally, but as soon as you focus on a different area where you acted immorally or hurt someone's feelings, then you will go back to 'feeling' bad about yourself. By contrast, if you accept yourself unconditionally, you will feel bad or good about your behaviour, but not bad or good about yourself on the basis of your behaviour.

If you would like to know more about developing self-acceptance, then I suggest that you consult my book on the subject entitled *How to Accept Yourself* (Sheldon Press, 1999).

Accept that you don't have to live up to your high moral expectations of yourself

If you are particularly prone to guilt, then it is likely that you will have high moral expectations of yourself – higher than you have for other people. It is a feature of people who are prone to guilt that they are much more accepting of others for behaviour that they would not tolerate in themselves. However, the real problem here is not the high standards of moral rectitude that you set for yourself. It is your rigid belief that you must achieve those high standards and that, if you don't, the only explanation for your failure is your moral badness as a person.

In my experience, people with guilt proneness rarely respond well to being encouraged to 'lower their moral standards'. Indeed, even if they decided to lower their moral standards, they would still be vulnerable to guilt were they to fail to reach their lowered moral standards. This would be owing to the fact that they would hold rigid beliefs about having to achieve these lowered standards. Consequently, if you do have high standards for yourself in the moral realm, then the way to become less prone to guilt is to keep such standards in place, at least for the time being, and challenge your rigid belief that you must achieve such standards. If you truly develop a flexible belief about achieving such high moral standards, you will acknowledge that, no matter how important achieving your high standards is to you, there is, sadly, no law of the universe that decrees that you must achieve them. If you truly believe this, you will not conclude that your failure proves your moral badness, but will see it as a failure of a fallible human being trying to live up to his or her standards, a failure that needs to be understood and learned from.

This is a point that bears repetition. When you feel guilty, you are preoccupied with your moral badness and, as such, it is very difficult for you to step back and reflect objectively on the reasons for your bad behaviour. When you feel remorse, on the other hand, you recognize that your failure reflects your fallibility and this insight will help you to stand back and reflect objectively on the reasons for your moral lapse.

Developing a flexible attitude about achieving your moral standards will then help you to weigh up the pros and cons of lowering these standards. However, whether or not you decide to do so, it is important that you develop a flexible philosophy about achievement of your moral standards no matter how high (or low) they are.

Dealing with your safety-seeking measures to avoid guilt

People often use safety-seeking measures to protect themselves from threat when they experience anxiety. You may use similar measures to protect yourself from feeling guilty. Here is how this works from your perspective. You reason that since you feel guilty about (1) doing the wrong thing, (2) failing to do the right thing and (3) hurting people's feelings, you will take steps to avoid guilt by always doing the right thing and never hurting people's feelings. Taking this decision means that you will not take risks in life (in case you do the wrong thing or upset others, for example), always put others first (so that others are not upset) and go out of your way to get people to like you (again to ensure that you do not upset them).

However, this behaviour and the reasoning that leads you to take it are flawed and will only serve to perpetuate your chronic guilt. This is due to the fact that your guilt is based not on you (1) doing the wrong thing, (2) failing to do the right thing and (3) hurting people's feelings, but on your irrational beliefs about these three inferences. So, if you want to deal effectively with guilt you need to do the following: take healthy risks, put yourself first – again, in a healthy way – and stop going out of your way to get people to like you, and see what happens. You will probably find that people are not as upset as you think and that you have not broken any of your moral codes.

However, if as a result of your behaviour you do break one of your moral codes, fail to live up to them or upset others, then you can deal with such situations by holding a set of rational beliefs about them so that you feel healthy remorse and not unhealthy guilt about these consequences.

Why you feel guilty much of the time and how to deal with this

If you are particularly prone to guilt you will think that you often do the wrong thing, fail to do the right thing or hurt the feelings of others.

You do this because you hold the following belief, which I call a 'chronic guilt-based general irrational belief':

> Whenever I am involved, I must make sure that nothing bad happens or that others' feelings are not hurt. If I don't and bad things happen and others are upset then it is all my fault and I am a bad person.

You then take this belief to relevant situations and, even where your involvement is minimal, you think that you are at fault if there is a bad outcome. As a result, you constantly think that you are responsible for any negative outcomes that happen or might happen and end up by blaming yourself.

How to deal with chronic guilt

In order to deal with this chronic sense of guilt, you need to develop and apply an alternative general rational belief which protects you from such guilt:

> Whenever I am involved, I want to make sure that nothing bad happens or that others' feelings are not hurt, but I don't have to succeed in doing so. If I don't succeed and bad things happen and others are upset, then I will take the appropriate level of responsibility, assign appropriate responsibility to others and consider

the impact of situational factors. I will accept myself for failing to adhere to my code and for any hurt that I inadvertently cause.

Such a belief will lead you to think that you have broken your moral code, failed to adhere to the code or hurt someone's feelings only when there is clear evidence for making such an inference. When there is, you will feel remorse rather than guilt because you will be processing this with a specific rational belief.

How to examine the accuracy of your guilt-related inference if necessary

If you are still unsure whether you have broken your moral code, failed to live up to it or hurt someone's feelings, answer one or more of the following questions:

- How valid is my inference that that I broke my moral code (for example)?
- Would an objective jury agree that I broke my moral code? If not, what would the jury's verdict be?
- Is my inference that I broke my moral code realistic? If not, what is a more realistic inference?
- If I asked someone I could trust to give me an objective opinion about my inference that I broke my moral code, what would the person say to me and why? What inference would this person encourage me to make instead?
- If a friend had told me that she (in this case) had made the same inference about breaking her moral code in the same situation, what would I say to her about the validity of her inference and why? What inference would I encourage the person to make instead?

Identify the action and thinking tendencies based on your guilt-related irrational beliefs and develop a list of alternative healthy action and thinking tendencies based on your general remorse-related rational beliefs. Resolve to practise the latter and limit the former.

In Chapter 2, I emphasized the fact that when you hold guilt-related irrational beliefs these beliefs have an effect on the way that you subsequently tend to think and act. If you turn these tendencies into actualities then you strengthen your conviction in these irrational beliefs and make yourself more prone to experience guilt.

In Chapter 3, on the other hand, I stressed that when you hold remorse-related irrational beliefs these beliefs have a different, and more constructive, effect on the way that you subsequently tend to think and act. If you turn these tendencies into actualities then you strengthen your conviction in these rational beliefs and make yourself less prone to experience guilt.

Following on from the above, I suggest that you do the following:

1 Develop a list of the ways in which you tend to think and act once you feel guilt.
2 Be aware of times when you experience the tendency to think and act in the above ways and resist doing so. Instead, use these tendencies to go back to challenge the guilt-related irrational beliefs that spawned them.
3 Develop a list of the ways in which you would tend to think and act if you held remorse-related rational beliefs. These should be constructive alternatives to the thinking and action tendencies that you listed under (1) above.
4 Once you have challenged your guilt-related irrational beliefs and have begun to hold the rational alternatives to these beliefs, encourage yourself to think and act in ways that are consistent with the thinking and action tendencies that you listed under (3).

Thus, a powerful way of making yourself less prone to guilt is to hold rational beliefs at the same time as you think and act in ways that reinforce such beliefs. If you hold remorse-related rational beliefs but think and act in ways that are consistent with the guilt-related irrational beliefs, you will tend to go back to these beliefs and spoil the work that you are trying to do to make yourself less prone to guilt. Thus, guard against doing this.

Dealing with failure to practise healthy self-care

People who have a chronic problem with guilt find it very hard to practise healthy self-care. The reason for this is as follows. Healthy self-care involves you putting yourself first unless others' needs are truly more important than your own. People with a chronic guilt problem generally think that others' needs are more important than their own and that to put oneself first is being selfish, which if you have a chronic problem you will seek to avoid. Putting others first helps you both avoid considering yourself a bad person, if you do put yourself first, and feel virtuous.

How to practise healthy self-care

In order to practise healthy self-care, you need to do the following:

• Develop a healthy general rational belief that underpins the practise of healthy self-care (e.g. 'I am a fallible human being, and if I don't look after myself then nobody will. I am not a bad person if I put myself first even though doing this is uncomfortable').

- Put this into practice and rehearse shortened specific versions of this general rational belief before you take self-caring action, while you do so and after you have done so.

Recognize that this will feel very uncomfortable because it will be unfamiliar. However, if you tolerate this discomfort and keep acting in ways that are consistent with your healthy general rational belief, then this discomfort will subside and eventually practising healthy self-care will become the familiar position for you.

Develop a realistic view on the question 'Can you hurt the feelings of others?'

Throughout this book I have used terms such as 'hurting people's feelings'. I have done so because this is how people prone to guilt tend to think. When you think that you have hurt someone's feelings this is an inference and, as we have seen in this book, people's emotional problems are not largely determined by inferences alone but are largely determined by the irrational beliefs that they hold about these inferences. Thus, you don't feel guilty because you think you have hurt someone's feelings, you feel guilty because you hold an irrational belief about this inference. So, in order to deal with guilt, you need to assume temporarily that you did, in fact, hurt someone's feelings so that you can identify, and deal effectively with, your guilt-inducing irrational beliefs.

When you have done this and are looking back at the event with your rational mind, it is useful to consider the question: 'Can I, in reality, hurt the feelings of others?' From the perspective of Cognitive Behavioural Therapy (CBT) the answer is no. When a person feels hurt about someone's behaviour, she (in this case) does so because she holds an irrational belief about that person's behaviour. So when you say that you have hurt someone's feelings, you are working on the assumption that your behaviour directly makes the other person feel hurt. You are implying that her beliefs play no part in this, which is patently false. So, it is important that you don't take responsibility for the other person's feelings. That does not mean that you can treat another person badly, safe in the knowledge that you aren't responsible for her feelings. Far from it!

What I am suggesting is that, while you should not take responsibility for the feelings of others, you should take full responsibility for the way you treat others. However, taking full responsibility for your behaviour does not mean that you have to blame yourself if you do treat someone badly, for responsibility is not synonymous with blame. If you do treat someone badly, it is healthy for you to feel remorse, an emotion based on a rational belief which will help you to stand back and learn from the experience so you are less likely to act that way in future.

Developing and rehearsing a non-guilty world view

People develop views of the world as it relates to them that make it more or less likely that they will experience unhealthy negative emotions. The world views that render you vulnerable to guilt do so in a similar way to the chronic guilt-based general irrational belief discussed above (i.e. 'Whenever I am involved, I must make sure that nothing bad happens or others' feelings are not hurt. If I don't, then it is all my fault and I am a bad person'): by making you focus unduly on things you have done that you think are wrong, your failures to do the right thing and the hurt you think you have caused others. However, these guilt-based world views have this effect on you much more widely.

Table 10.1 World views that render you vulnerable to guilt and help you to deal with guilt

Views of the world that render you vulnerable to guilt	Views of the world that help you deal with guilt
Other people's desires are more important than my own.	My desires are no less important to me than others' desires are to them. I can flexibly and healthily prioritize my desires in the same way as others can flexibly and healthily prioritize theirs.
When I am involved I have responsibility for the hurt feelings of others.	When I am involved, I have responsibility for my actions, but ultimately I am not responsible for the feelings of others. They are.
In the moral domain, I expect more of myself than I do of others.	In the moral domain, I can expect the same of myself as I can expect of others.
It is possible to always act morally.	It is rarely possible to always act morally since if you do the right thing from one perspective you may be doing the wrong thing from another perspective.
Saying no to others is a sign of selfishness.	Saying no to others may be selfish, but is more likely to be a sign of healthy self-care.

It is important that you develop realistic views of the world that will help you to deal with guilt. In Table 10.1, you will find an illustrative list of such world views rather than an exhaustive one, to give you an idea of what I mean so that you can develop your own. In Table 10.1, I first describe a world view that renders you vulnerable to guilt and then I give its healthy alternative. You will see that the latter is characterized by the idea that you are as important and as fallible as others, whereas in the former you are less important and more responsible than others.

If you hold rational beliefs that are consistent with the views of the world listed on the right-hand side of Table 10.1 and if you act and think in ways that are, in turn, consistent with these rational beliefs, then doing all this will help you become less prone to guilt.

This brings us to the end of the book. If you would like to offer me any feedback, please write to me c/o the publisher.

Index

ABC framework
  chronic guilt and 23
  dealing with vulnerability 91–2
  other people's beliefs 36
  outline of 1–6
  remorse and 26–7
  strengthening rational beliefs
    86–8
  see also adversity; beliefs,
  irrational; beliefs, rational;
  consequences
acceptance
  about life 98
  meaning of 4
  remorse and 26–7
  see also self-acceptance
adversity (A)
  ABC model 4
  assessing your guilt 62–3
  context of guilt 52
  guilt versus remorse 25, 39
  meaning of 2, 4
  rational-emotive imagery 82
amends, making 31–2
anger with self 47
anxiety 106–7
assertiveness
  healthy self-care 109–10
  non-guilty world view 111
  standing up for yourself 21–2,
    35
attack–response technique 78–81
awfulizing
  meaning of 3
  non-awfulizing 4
  about relapse 97, 98

Beck, Dr Aaron 1
behaviour
  assessing the context of 29–30
  assessing your guilt 60
  based on irrational beliefs 16–19
  defining your problem 49
  guilt versus remorse 39

meaning of 5
rational beliefs 30–2, 84–6
setting goals 52–3, 61
beliefs (B), irrational
  challenging 103–4
  chronic guilt and 20–3
  guilt-based 8–13, 34
  guilt versus remorse 39
  hurting others' feelings 110–11
  identifying 63–4
  imagery method 81–2
  outline of ABC model 2–4
  part–whole error 74–5
  questioning yourself 65–77
  refraining from 86
  thinking that stems from 13–16
  true or false 69–70
  types of 2–3
beliefs (B), rational
  attack–response 78–81
  behaviour stemming from 30–2
  developing 104
  guilt versus remorse 39
  identifying 64
  preventing relapse 90
  questioning yourself 65–77
  rehearsing actions and thinking
    84–6
  about relapse 96–9
  self-care and 109–10
  self-statements 83–4
  strengthen your conviction
    78–86
  teaching others 83
  thinking based on 28
  true or false 69–70
  underpinning remorse 26–8

Cognitive Behavioural Therapy
  (CBT)
  focus of 1
  other people's feelings 110
  see also Rational Emotive
  Behaviour Therapy (REBT)

compassion 15
confession 16
consequences (C)
    ABC model 5
    assessing your response 59–61
    meaning of 2, 5–6
    setting goals for remorse 52–6
    see also behaviour; emotions;
        thinking
cost–benefit analysis of guilt 40–6

depreciation, self-
    attack–response 80
    deserving/undeserving conflict
        11
    for having guilt 46–7
    identifying 63–4
    meaning of 3
    over-generalizing 9
    proneness to guilt 102
    questioning 72–7
    selflessness/selfish conflict
        10–11
depriving yourself 17
discomfort in/tolerance
    meaning of 3, 4
    relapse and 97

Ellis, Dr Albert 1, 2
emotions
    assessing your guilt 60
    dealing with guilt problems
        101–2
    defining healthy/unhealthy 5
    setting goals 61
    setting realistic goals and 52
Epictetus 1, 2
exaggerated thinking 13

factors of the situation
    all the data 28–9, 62
    complexity of 15–16
    describing 58–9
    mitigating 15, 29, 62
flexible beliefs 3
    identifying 64
    questioning 67–72, 70–2
    about relapse 96, 98
    remorse and 26

forgiveness
    accepting offers of 32
    asking for 30–1
    begging for 17
    rejecting offers of 19
goals
    realistic remorse 52–6
    three components 61–2
guilt
    accepting your proneness to
        102
    accuracy of your inferences
        108–9
    acknowledging problem of
        100–1
    analysis of dis/advantages of
        40–5
    assessing your problem 37–40,
        57–64
    being versus feeling 7
    chronic 20–3, 40, 107–8
    compared to remorse 38–40
    defining your problem with
        48–9
    identifying patterns of 103
    making inferences 7–8
    non-guilty world view 111–12
    safety-seeking to avoid 106–7
    setting realistic goals 52–6
    working on episode of 102–3
    your vulnerability to 90–6

harming others/hurting feelings
    assessing your situation 62–3
    describing your problem 51–2
    inferences about 8, 25
    realistic view of 110
    remorse 28
    setting goals for remorse 55–6
hindsight judgement 15

'if only' thinking 14–15
imagery *see* rational-emotive
    imagery

making excuses 32
manipulation by others 21, 35
Maultsby Jr, Dr Maxie C. 47

meta-disturbances 101
mitigating factors 15, 29, 62
moral codes
    acts of commission 49–50, 53–4
    acts of omission 50–1, 54–5
    assessing your situation 62–3
    breaking 8, 11–12, 25
    complexity of humans 104–5
    failing to live up to 8, 12, 25
    harming others 8, 12–13
    high self-expectation and
        105–6
    inferences about 8
    rational beliefs about 27–8
    self-expectation 111
    setting realistic goals 52–5

National Institute for Health and
    Clinical Excellence (NICE) 1

overcompensation 18–19

penance 18
promises 17
psychopaths 36
punishment
    atonement with penalty 31
    expectation of 16
    penalty versus retribution 30
    self- 17–18

Rational Emotive Behaviour
    Therapy (REBT) 2–6
    see also ABC framework
rational-emotive imagery 81–2
    of constructive behaviour 93–5
    preventing relapse 92–3
rational self-statements 83–4
reassurance
    asking forgiveness and 17
    seeking 19
relapse prevention
    rational beliefs about 96–9
    reviewing your achievements
        89, 95–6
    thinking through situations 89
    your vulnerability 90–3
remorse
    alternative to guilt 24

for clear 'sin' 32–5
    commitment to 66–7, 101
    compared to guilt 38–40
    disadvantages of 45–6
    dynamics of 24
    as healthy alternative 101
    independence from
        manipulation 35
    inferences 25
    pain from realization 30
    rational beliefs 26–32
    rational-emotive imagery 82
    setting goals and 53–6
    see also beliefs, rational
responsibility
    appropriate levels of 29
    assuming too much 14
    for a clear 'sin' 33
    disclaiming 18
    for others' feelings 22–3, 36,
        110–11
    setting realistic goal 62
rigid beliefs 2–3
    characteristics of 67
    defining 9
    identifying 63–4
    questioning 67–72

self-acceptance 46–7
    falling from 'grace' 104–5
    high moral code and 105–6
    identifying rational beliefs 64
    questioning 72–7
    relapse and 97
self-care
    healthy 109–10
self-control 97
selflessness/selfishness
    conflict of 10–11
    inferences of situation 58–9
    non-guilty world view 111
    self-care 22, 35–6

thinking
    assessing your guilt 60–1
    based on rational beliefs 28–30
    guilt versus remorse 39
    from irrational beliefs 13–16
    meaning of 5–6

rehearsing rational beliefs 84–6
setting goal 62
wrongdoing
clear 'sin' 32–5

understanding reasons for 31

zigzag technique (attack–response)
78–81